TEA CLEANSE DIET

How to Choose Your Detox Teas, Lose Weight and Improve
Health

(How to Choose Your Detox Teas, Boost Your Metabolism)

Dana Mason

Published by Sharon Lohan

© Dana Mason

Tea Cleanse Diet: How to Choose Your Detox Teas, Lose Weight and Improve Health (How to Choose Your Detox Teas, Boost Your Metabolism)

ISBN 978-1-990334-38-2

Legal & Disclaimer

The information contained in this book is not designed to replace or take the place of any form of medicine or professional medical advice. The information in this book has been provided for educational and entertainment purposes only.

Table of contents

PART 1

INTRODUCTION

Anyone who's ever struggled with weight loss knows just how hard it can be to get rid of all that excess flab. We are all well aware of just how important is to follow a healthy diet and exercise regimen, but these things are easier said than done.

People who have completely restructured their lifestyles can attest to the fact that doing so almost always involves giving up on foods, habits and routines that are integral to your life. There's also the matter of making all that effort to cook the right foods and make time for the gym. And because the results take so long to start showing that it can be really hard to find the motivation to stick it out. And so, most weight loss programs and resolutions fail before they even really have a chance to take off.

What if you could lose all that unwanted weight without having to try your luck with fad diets and grueling workout programs? What if you could lose weight without needing to follow any challenging diets or spending hours sweating it out in the gym? What if you no longer needed to spend months squinting at the mirror checking to see if you look any different yet? What if all you have to do was and a cup of tea or two to your diet?

That's right. With the help of this e-book and the secrets of tea cleansing, you're going to be able to lose more weight than ever before. It's easy, fast, healthy and completely foolproof!

Read on to begin with your weight loss journey!

CHAPTER 1: ALL ABOUT THAT BREW

The world is divided into two kinds of people: the tea drinkers and the coffee drinkers. Yes, there is a population of people that avoid both beverages for health reasons, but by the end of this e-book we are pretty sure they'll be rooting for the tea team!

Most people can't do without their morning cuppa. You might have tried to go without it for a few days but you'll find yourself feeling tired, cranky, lethargic and just so slow. The morning cup slowly, but surely, evolves into a few more through the day and as a result, most people are warned about staying off these beverages altogether. For most tea and coffee lovers, it becomes a lifelong struggle defined by periods of complete abstinence followed by periods of complete dependency. It doesn't sound pretty, but what if there was a way around the negative effects of your daily beverage needs and your fat loss challenges without any sacrifices? What if you could combine the two into one spectacular solution? Sounds impossible, right? It's not!

In this e-book we are going to study the power of the tea cleanse. You are probably wondering how something as delicious and indulgent as tea could possibly constitute a cleanse. Well, it does. And this e-book is going to teach you all about it.

Now, for the coffee lovers who are wondering where all this talk of tea leaves them, we have some substitutes for you as well. Unfortunately, a coffee cleanse really is a far-fetched notion and most people already know that the health risks of a coffee addiction are far greater than the minimal benefits (if any) the beverage offers. This e-book does include some tea substitutes that have been known to appeal to most coffee lovers, so hopefully you will be able to pick up some new dietary preferences there. And of course, at the end of the day, it is about losing that weight and getting to a place where you look and feel good. Switching from coffee to a healthy tea is certainly worth the result. The good thing about tea is that there are so many different variants and most of them are pretty healthy in the original forms. It's just a matter of learning how to combine them and making sure you drink them in a form that's healthy and conducive to your weight goals.

Let us begin with a little background and some interesting tidbits about tea.

Simply the mention of the word "tea" immediately invokes images of delicate porcelain cups and saucers, lush green fields, hot steaming cups of chai, as the spicy, milky variant is known, and more. The beautiful thing about tea is its universal appeal: all sorts of cultural borders and geographical limits dissolve into that little whirlpool you hold between your palms.

The discovery of tea can be traced back to China around 2737 BC, but the exact historical facts have gotten lost over the ages and this wondrous beverage has woven its way into legends and narratives as refreshing as the drink itself. In China, tea has long been a staple with both the ruling classes and the common folk for the numerous medicinal and herbal benefits it offers. In the Western Zhou Dynasty, tea played an instrumental role as an offering during religious ceremonies. The famed Han Dynasty experienced a shortage of tea plants and so; the consumption of tea was a luxury of the wealthy and the blue-blooded alone. It was in the Tang Dynasty that more varieties of the plant were unearthed and drinking tea became a truly egalitarian practice. The popularization of tea saw endorsements by the government and lots of little teashops springing up everywhere.

Soon, the beverage found its way to Japan by way of the priests who were located in China for their education and training. Initially limited to the priests, tea in Japanese culture slowly permeated through to the Buddhist community in general and then further on to the rest of the population.

Most people, especially in the Western world, associate the practice of drinking tea with the English. The plant and the beverage were, in fact, introduced to England in the 17th century. Established as the beverage of the royals, tea quickly became the symbol of status and luxury and the good life amongst the English upper society. Tea has historically grown wonderfully in the fertile fields of India. The East India Company exported tea to Britain, where the taxes on the 'luxury beverage' were so high that the East India Company also turned to America to draw in greater revenue.

And so, this elixir-like beverage found its way all around the world.

DIFFERENT TYPES OF TEA

Don't worry; we're going to come to the good stuff real soon. But learning more about tea definitely helps in understanding the role it has to play in your nutritional intake and gets us once step closer to understanding how tea can be used to quick-start fat loss. We're now going to take a look at the different types of tea available. These vary in terms of ingredients, brewing/ preparation requirements, appearances, tastes and most importantly, health benefits.

You could simply go out and buy yourself a detox tea plan and spend a whole lot of money and not bother with all this information. Or, you can learn all there is to know about teas and then make your own, informed choices. To suit your body type, health requirements and weight loss plans. Now, which sounds better? An expensive, one-size-fits-all readymade detox program or a carefully created tea cleanse that's got everything that YOU need? The latter, right? Thought so! Read on to learn more about the different types of teas.

Green Teas

If you've ever trying to lose weight knowing you've got a tea habit, someone or the other must have recommended Green tea to you at some point. It's not just a health fad: Green tea contains an antioxidant compound called catechin.

Green teas are not oxidized, which is why they are able to retain the telltale color (though it's not always a true green; the color can vary between a pale lemony yellow and a deep green). The leaves are processed with heat to remove any traces of the enzyme that causes oxidation. Every leaf responds to the heat treatment differently, and as a result, the flavor varies from batch-to-batch and even leaf-to-leaf.

A specific kind of Green tea, the Matcha tea, is currently the darling of the health-conscious world. The frothy, bright green tea is not only a delight to look at, but also really good for the body.

Black Teas

Black tea contains some of the highest levels of caffeine in any tea: we are talking about as much 40mg of caffeine for every standard cup. So, if you're looking for a healthier alternative to your daily cup of coffee, black tea is the way to go. It's healthier because it contains theaflavins and thearubigins, both of which are antioxidants that are known to help control cholesterol spikes in the body.

Black teas have a distinctively smoky flavor to them, but are also often laced with a honey-like taste. Black teas are very popular with those who prefer tea 'blends' instead of a single, dominant tea ruling the cup. Blending allows for creating a myriad of flavors and strengths, and so there is a black tea for every taste and occasion.

The Darjeeling and the Lapsang Souchong are possibly the most well known Black teas around the world.

White Teas

White teas are also rich in catechins, much like Green teas.

White teas are a great option if you want a tea that undergoes the most minimal processing. The tealeaves are generally just steamed and then allowed to dry. They are the least processed variant on this entire list.

The cultivation of this particular variant of tealeaves is limited to only a handful of days around the entire year. The leaf pickers wait until a white down appears on the shoots of the tea plant and that is when they pick the leaves. White teas are some of the most exclusive teas available because the cultivation, the drying and all other stages of the preparatory process require time, attention and an exact knowledge on part of the tea makers.

Belonging to the floral bouquets class of teas, White teas have a very delicate flavor and aroma. Most tea enthusiasts will find that the flavors of White teas invoke likenesses to the essences of bamboo and almonds.

One of the most popular and most sought-after types of White tea is the Silver Needle: it is manufactured using just the most tender of the white, downy shoots and has the most unsullied flavor imaginable.

Oolong Teas

Oolong is particularly good for people trying to lose weight because this type of tea triggers enzymes that help decrease the presence of triglycerides (a particular kind of fat) in the blood. A known fat burner, Oolong is also chockfull of niacin and antioxidants, both of which are great for when you are looking for a detox and want to cleanse your body of any and all impurities.

Oolong teas follow under the category of teas that are semi-oxidized. The teas are made using the bigger, mature leaves. These are allowed to wither and rolled before they are oxidized and then fire-treated.

Oolong contains a smaller dose of caffeine as compared to Black teas and Green teas. In general, the caffeine levels will depend upon the brewing method and time.

The taste and character of the Oolong will change with the time/ repetitions of steeping. Unlike many other types of teas, the Oolong responds well to prolonged and repetitive steeping, treating you to a new texture and taste every time.

Pu'erh Teas

Pu'erh teas are a type of fermented teas that are traced to the Pu'erh town in China. Research has shown that Pu'erh teas can help the digestion process and also help control cholesterol levels in the body, thus making them a welcome addition to weight loss programs.

The tea leaves are usually compressed and then aged for a long time, during which period they can be treated to bacteria and microflora that contribute to the fermentation process much like in the case of wine. The older the leaves, the more exclusive the tea is considered to be. And if there's one universal feature of markets the world over, it is that the more exclusive a product is the more expensive it will be.

The brew from Pu'erh leaves is dark and contains a minimal amount of caffeine, and offers the drinker a subtle, earthy flavor.

Herbal Teas

Herbal teas are some of the healthiest kids around this block; there is no end to the different concoctions that you can brew up and every herb offers its own health benefits and has a different role to play in terms of weight loss. The great thing about herbal teas is that not only do you get your much-needed daily dose of energy; you also get to cash in on all sorts of immunity-boosting and body-strengthening health benefits that you might not be able to work into the rest of your diet. Lemon teas, ginger teas, chamomile teas etc. are only some of the great herbal teas that offer all kinds of natural health benefits, are bursting to the brim with antioxidants and pack a wallop against fat deposits.

Herbal infusions are prepared with all sorts of natural ingredients, including floral and herbal elements. Apart from the significant health benefits they offer, herbal teas are also popular because of the exciting colors, aromas and flavors: this makes them a rather welcome addition to any diet.

Herbal teas generally contain little to no caffeine, but nonetheless have an energizing and refreshing effect on the body. As such, they're not harsh at all and let you enjoy the benefits of tea without posing any risks to your health. We're going to take a look at some specific kinds of herbal-infused brews later in this e-book as well.

Mate Teas

Remember when we said that there would be some great options in here especially geared towards meeting the needs of coffee lovers? Well, Mate teas are well known as a favorite substitute for those who generally like their daily dose of energy from caffeine instead.

These teas are a derivative of the South American yerba mate plant and are available in a variety of flavors, strengths, herbal infusions, spices and more.

Mate teas are also available as teabags that contain a mixture of the Mate leaves, a little bit of coffee and some spices for added flavor. While this e-book is dedicated to helping you lose weight with the help of cleansing your body with tea alone, this particular option might appeal to you if you are having a particularly hard time making the switch.

HEALTH BENEFITS OF DRINKING TEA

If the scrumptious teas discussed in the previous section have you longing for a cup right now, go ahead and brew one! Just be sure to come back and learn about the various health benefits of drinking tea.

Before you embark on a tea cleanse, it is important to learn about the different ways in which tea affects your body. The entire point of the tea cleanse, and this e-book, is to shed unwanted weight fast. But that doesn't mean that you can't look forward to other health benefits along the way. That is exactly what is so great about making tea a part of your diet: it helps target so many different health concerns and works on so many different levels.

We'll get to the weight loss in just a moment, but till then, here are some of the other reasons why drinking tea is such a great idea:

1. Remember how we discussed that Green tea contains the antioxidant catechin? Catechin is a source of EGCG and it is said that the same may help fortify the body against heart disease and malignancy.
2. Most types of tea contain antioxidants in varying quantities. The thing about antioxidants is that they act like a shield. Imagine an invisible layer guarding your body against all kinds of infections and strengthening it from the inside out. That is what antioxidants do.
3. And while antioxidants aren't magic and can't quite reverse the fact or effects of ageing, they certainly slow down the negative impact of it. You continue to look and feel younger for much longer than people who don't incorporate healthy teas into their lifestyle.

4. The EGCG found in Green tea is being studied for its potential in preventing the onset of neurological diseases like Parkinson's disease and Alzheimer's.

Remember how we talked about the endless possibilities and potential of herbal teas? Well, here's one that gives you some food for thought: Chamomile tea contains antioxidants that can help you battle against some of the debilitating health problems that arise from diabetes, such as kidney damage, nerve damage and deteriorating vision.

5. Research has shown that teas contain active compounds that fight inflammation and ease swelling and other aggravated reactions to most injuries, illnesses, conditions and psychosomatic ailments. Anyone who has ever experienced inflammation related to arthritis or depression will know just how painful and difficult it can be to live with. So, a cup of tea won't just help lift your spirits, it will actually help ease the pain and the cause of it!
6. The antioxidants in tea also help battle the harmful effects of pollution. We've already talked about how antioxidants act as a protective layer against all kinds of health issues: well, they do the same against problems caused by pollution. Some of the common adverse effects of pollution like damaged skin, brittle hair and respiratory ailments are

effectively tackled by the antioxidants present in tea.

7. Tea contains polyphenols and these have been linked to stronger immunity against cancers of various kinds. Medicinal science is yet to conclusively verify the claim that tea can help prevent cancer but exhaustive research has shown a definite trend in support of the same. Tea drinkers have reported fewer malignancies and vulnerabilities as compared to those who do not partake of the beverage, and this particular phenomenon has been attributed to the presence of polyphenols in tea.

8. Tea is known for its excellent oxygen radical absorbance capacity. Why is this important? Because it helps target the DNA-harming free radicals in the body. Even though the body is supposed to deal with free radicals on its own, it can miss some of them every now and then. That's where tea comes in handy. As a result, it helps to stave off several debilitating diseases such as neurological collapse, cardiovascular diseases and other degenerative conditions.

9. Research has established that consuming Green tea can help to build the mineral density as well as the general overall health of your bones. This can go a long way in prevent injuries, fatigue and orthopedic ailments.

10. The polyphenols found in tea have also been linked to helping brain functions like learning, information retention and clarity of memory and connection work well. That is one of the reasons why tea is said to help prevent diseases like Alzheimer's. This property of tea also makes it beneficial for people who have trouble with focusing, attentiveness, alertness, absorbing information and remembering it over extended periods of time without the presence of a neurological disease.

11. Black tea has been known to help fortify the lungs against the damaging effects of cigarette smoke. This does not mean you should take up smoking as a habit, or continue it if you already are a smoker and just try even things out by adding some black tea to your diet! But if you have been exposed to cigarette smoke or are worried about regularly inhaling second-hand smoke, apart from limiting your exposure to it you can also consume black tea to mitigate some of the effects on your respiratory system.

These are just some of the many, many ways in which your body stands to benefit from drinking tea. It is quite astonishing to realize that an innocuous little cup could do so much for you. And to think, a lot of people would have recommended giving up the habit altogether!

The truth is that you need to be able to strike a balance and not cross over from healthy regular consumption, to a 10-milk-and-sugar-cups-a-day addiction.

LOSING WEIGHT WITH TEA: BOOST METABOLISM, LOOSE FAT

Now we come to the good stuff: using a tea cleanse program to get rid of excess weight and unwanted flab. Before we dive into the specific recipes and your 15-day tea cleanse weight loss program, let us take a look at how tea helps us to lose weight.

The reason why a tea cleanse forms the heart of our weight loss program is because it helps to jumpstart weight loss on two fundamental levels: it helps increase your natural metabolism and helps your body cut fat. In doing so, not only is it making your body more receptive to efforts like dieting and exercising but also working actively to get rid of any pudginess. As a result, the tea cleanse works both on the inside and the outside!

Different teas will offer you different benefits as part of a tea cleanse. You can choose to incorporate the teas that are most useful for achieving your specific goals or you can follow the 15-day program to lose as much as 10 pounds in 15 days.

Let's take a look at how teas can help you lose weight the healthy way.

1 We're back with yet another benefit of Green tea. Remember catechin? Looks like the antioxidant is just full of one benefit after the other. We all know that antioxidants are really good for the body because they help detox. The antioxidants also help flush out impurities from the body and stimulate weight and fat loss. If you've ever wondered why all your dietary and exercise efforts aren't making a difference, it is because the body will usually respond for a little bit before it plateaus. And the toxins accumulated in the body over time will work against all your efforts. So, sometimes you need to just completely clean out the body of all the impurities before you can start building up the good. That's where the concept of the tea cleanse comes in, and that is why the antioxidants from tea are necessary to any weight loss plan.

2 Oolong tea is the one that is most recommended for people trying to lose weight. If you want to do the tea cleanse to lose 10 pounds in 15 days, making Oolong tea a part of your diet is a very good idea. In fact, Wuyi, a specific type of Oolong tea is rather popular as a weight loss supplement. What makes Oolong such a hit with folks looking to lose weight and cut fat? Oolong helps to energize an enzyme that helps destroy triglycerides. These are a kind of

dietary fat that get deposited in the fat cells in the body.

3   As a result of its fat-burning properties, Oolong tea helps achieve a higher calorie burn than normal. A study was used to observe women who consume Oolong tea as compared to those who do not. It was found that over two-hour periods of observation, women who did drink Oolong burned a higher number of calories at the same activity level as compared to women who do not.

4   Do you know what is responsible for that layer of fat around your stomach? Anyone who has ever tried to lose weight and tone up knows that belly fat is the hardest to get rid off: it just refuses to budge! Well, that specific area is usually affected by cortisol, which is the hormone that the body releases in times of stress and anxiety. The cortisol hormone creates fat deposits along the tummy and once they're there, getting rid of them can be a real challenge. Luckily for you, this tea cleanse can make that seemingly impossible goal a breeze! Tea is known to reduce cortisol levels in the body, which means that you're going to have fewer and fewer fat deposits to complain of. Even when you do experience some stress, consuming tea regularly helps prevent cortisol levels from shooting up. Not only does tea prevent cortisol levels from rising, it also targets the effect that cortisol has on the body: this means that the existing quantities of cortisol

will not result in fat/ weight gain if you make healthy teas a part of your regular diet.

5   Pu-erh tea is another kind of tea that has been linked to weight loss. Research has indicated that Pu-erh tea might help prevent weight gain, while also working actively to lower the levels of LDL cholesterol in the body. As such, you are looking at a slimmer, fitter you in no time!

6   Everyone knows that a high metabolism rate can really help boost weight loss while a low metabolism rate is basically a death knell for any fitness plans you might have. If you suffer from a poor metabolic rate, you'll have to put in twice (maybe even thrice) the amount of effort into exercising and dieting to lose the most minimal amount of weight and fat. It just isn't fair! Well, let's tip the scales in your favor the, shall we? Tea is known to boost natural metabolism rates, thereby helping you achieve a higher calorie burn than usual. In fact, Green tea is the best for this purpose: the simple act of drinking it fives times everyday can help you burn 80 extra calories! Imagine burning calories, losing weight and cutting fat while drinking tea. Do you know what this means in the long run? This kind of burn, spread out of a year, could help you lose anywhere between eight and ten pounds, while doing nothing strenuous or uncomfortable!

7 Tea by itself contains little to no calories. People who complain of putting on weight as a result of a tea habit need to dig a little deeper into their dietary preferences to trace the actual root of the evil. More often than not, the weight gain is actually a result of the body's response to the added milk/dairy supplements that a lot of people take with their tea. And, of course, there is always the case of all that added sugar: that will pack on the pounds like nothing else. Try going dairy-free with your tea and watch the pounds just melt off. If you need a little sweetener, skip the sugar and the artificial sweeteners and go the more natural route with honey. It still means some calorific intake but it comes with an added boost of healthy nutrients.

8 Research has shown that people who consume hot tea regularly are able to maintain a lower BMI in the long run, as compared to people who don't drink tea. So, you're looking at an overall reduction in size, weight and fat!

9 A study focusing on people who drink hot tea on a daily basis and those that do not found that the latter usually suffer from a larger waist circumference on an average. That means that drinking tea might actually help you keep your girth in check!

10 Catcechin (does the potential of this little miracle-worker ever cease?) also helps the body use up the stored fat deposits as much-needed fuel during exercise. This way, you're getting twice the usual benefits with your workout: the calorific burn as of itself and the accumulated fat is ripped right off. This fat-as-fuel burn actually helps increase muscle strength and stamina, letting you exercise for longer and burn more calories.

11 One of the benefits of drinking Green tea is that it is supposed to help people living with Type 2 Diabetes process sugars in a more improved manner and at a better rate. While this is certainly great news for people with Type 2 Diabetes, if you don't have the disease but would still like to gain from the benefits of this property of Green tea, there's nothing stopping you! Sugars in small quantities might not do much damage to the body but you'd be surprised at how much sugar exists in the food and beverages we consume daily. Even foods you wouldn't typically think of as 'sugary' can contain high quantities of sugar. So, making sure that it is processed properly, absorbed well and then expended thoroughly is of the utmost importance to those looking to lose weight. Luckily, it seems like the only thing you need to be able to kick start this particular goal of yours is just a little bit of Green tea

12   We're building up a little on the facts we discussed in point #4 regarding cortisol and weight gain here. In the year 2006 a research was conducted, analyzing the dietary habits and related weight loss/gain experiences of people with a view to interpret the role played by tea in the same. It was found that people who consume tea every day might experience the same kind of stressors as those who do not, and might indeed have a similar emotional/ psychological reaction to the trigger but did not actually share a physiological response. The cortisol levels in people who do drink tea was decidedly low and even people who were given placebos to check for veracity did not display such a marked decrease in stress-response-cortisol-release. It was found that those experiencing lower levels of cortisol invariably experienced a slimming-down of the mid-section as well as anti-ageing effects!

CHAPTER 2: TERRIFIC TEAS – RECIPES TO TRY TODAY!

So we've covered all the reasons why a tea cleanse is just the thing you need to lose those last 10 pounds. Stubborn as those can be, they are no match for the tea detox options in this e-book. In this chapter, we're going to take a look at three genius tea recipes that are absolutely ruthless against those pesky fat deposits and unwanted blips on the weighing skills.

Try one (or more!) of these today to figure out which one suits you best!

#1 GARLIC AND GREEN

This is hands-down the winner of all fat loss teas out there, and it is so easy to make. The recipe is probably the world's worst kept fitness secret, and once you start seeing results you'll wonder how you hadn't already heard of it.

Ingredients:

- 1 Green teabag
- 3 cloves of garlic- sliced in half
- ½ tbsp. lemon juice- freshly squeezed
- ½ tbsp. honey- or to taste
- 1 ½ cups of water

Preparation:

1. Add water and garlic pieces to a saucepan. Let the mix boil.
2. Turn the flame off. Add the lemon juice. Add the honey.
3. Add the teabag.
4. Let the mixture steep for 5 minutes.
5. Remove the teabag. Strain the mixture to remove garlic pieces.
6. Wait until the tea is no longer boiling hot.
7. Sip while warm.

#2 Icy Green To Get Hot While Staying Cool

Why should all teas be enjoyed hot? No reason why you can't get the amazing weight loss benefits of Green tea and keep it cool this summer! Here's an icy cool recipe for when the temperature's soaring and your weight isn't the only thing you want to lower!

Ingredients:

- 1 Green teabag
- 3-4 whole strawberries- finely diced
- ½ lemon- freshly squeezed
- ¼- ½ cucumber- finely chopped
- 1 ½ cup water
- ½ 1tbsp. honey

Preparation:

- Add water to a saucepan. Bring to a boil. Switch the heat off.
- Add the teabag. Allow it to steep for 5 minutes. Remove the teabag.
- Let the brew cool.
- Add the strawberries, lemon juice and cucumber pieces to a blender.
- Add the honey.
- Add the tea brew.
- Blend until properly combined.
- Refrigerate tea to chill.
- Serve cold.

#3 SMOOTHIE TEA

Smoothies are a favorite with health-conscious folks all over the world. If you enjoy smoothies, you can now pack in even more of a punch with some added green tea. Whoever thought something like a smoothie tea could be real? But it is! And it is yum, full of the goodness of citrus fruits and an excellent dietary addition for when you need some extra strength (maybe for a workout?) but also want all the slimming benefits of tea.

Ingredients:

- 1 grapefruit
- 1 orange
- ½ lemon squeezed
- ½ banana- frozen
- ½ cup Greek yogurt- low fat/ nonfat variety
- ½ cup of prepared Green tea, cooled
- 1 cup ice
- ½ tbsp. honey

Preparation:

1 Prepare some Green tea and let it cool. Then refrigerate it to chill it. Don't add any sweeteners.
2 Peel and slice the fruits and add them to the blender.
3 Add the yogurt.
4 Add the Green tea.

5 Add the honey.
6 Blend till it's all mixed.
7 Add the ice and blend again. Make sure the ice is properly crushed and you're not left over with any bits to chew on!
8 Serve!

You can always add the zest of a citrusy fruit for some extra garnishing. You might also want to increase/reduce the amount of honey depending on how sweet you like your tea.

Chapter 3: Your 15 – Day Fat Loss Program

Now, for those of you who have been waiting for a surefire way to drop 10 pounds in 15 days, here is our secret tea cleanse. This 15-day fat loss program is going to detox the body and shred that fat like you wouldn't believe. Here's everything you need to know about the tea cleanse fat loss program!

Now, we've already shared three exciting tea cleanse recipes to get your fat loss program off to a roaring start. One cup of each of these per day is going to get your body ready to start dropping those pounds pronto!

We're also going to take a look at three special teas that form the core of the 15-day fat loss program. You might think that six cups of tea throughout the day might be a bit much, but don't forget: these are all-natural recipes without any of the gunky processed foods, heavy dairy and artificial sugars. There's nothing but fat-melting, body-blasting goodness in these cups.

If you're not keen on hitting the ground running and you want to build it up with baby-steps, use the three teas discussed in this chapter as part of your 15-day fat loss program and slowly start including the three recipes discussed in the previous chapter as you develop a taste for the teas- and a desire to see more of the incredible weight loss you are going to experience in no time at all.

The reason why these teas are not only allowed, but also in fact recommended in such quantities is because they contain all kinds of healthy, immunity-and-endurance-boosting ingredients that also help you fight fat. None of the ingredients are going to harm your body in any way or cause you to gain weight. If you paid attention in the previous chapter you will have noticed that none of the teas called for adding milk or sugar. That's why they're so healthy: they not only incorporate the best of what Nature has to offer but also do away with anything that could get in the way of your weight loss goals.

And finally, you should always allow yourself some room for adaptation to suit your personal tastes and weight loss goals. We've got recommendations on the when and how, but listen to your body and adapt if you need to!

FAT LOSS TEA #1

Now, this one's a somewhat more complex brew than all the others listed in this e-book, and the ingredients might require a little hunting and gathering on your part. But the results are stupendous. We're talking a smaller waist, increased metabolism, lowered water retention and clear skin right away! And this one's the only tough one in the tea cleanse. Promise!

Ingredients:

- 2 parts eleuthero root
- 2 parts nettle leaves
- 1 cup water
- 1 part dandelion leaf/ ½ tsp. dried dandelion
- 1 part papaya leaf
- 1 part senna leaf
- 1 part slippery elm bark
- 1 part marshmallow root
- ½ part ginger root
- ½ part cinnamon bark
- ½ part orange peel
- ¼ part fennel seeds

Preparation:

1 Add all the ingredients to a bowl and mix well.
2 Take the water in a saucepan and bring to a boil.

3 Add the mixed ingredients to the water and let it simmer. Wait until the mix infuses well with the water. Simmer another minute.
4 Turn the flame off.
5 Let it steep.
6 Cool a bit and sip warm.

Expert Advice:

You can also consume this tea cool, and since preparing it is a bit of a fiddly task, why not brew up a batch and sip it through the day or store some for the next day? Make sure you have at least a cup a day, and time it for early evening.

Fat Loss Tea #3 – Lose With Lemon

Look, we just can't get enough of lemony teas. They're zingy, they're energizing, they help fortify the body and they are just the best for weight loss. The cinnamon powder will help you control your blood sugar levels and will keep hunger at bay. The cayenne pepper is known to be a fat-burner, as is lemon itself. This particular infusion also battles salt cravings and sweet cravings, and helps keep your body hydrated.

Ingredients:

- ½ lemon- sliced in fourths, with the peel
- ¼ tsp. apple cider vinegar (start out with an eight of a teaspoon to figure out your own tastes first)
- 1/16 tsp. or 1 pinch cayenne pepper
- 1 tsp. honey
- 1/16 tsp. or 1 pinch cinnamon powder
- 1½ cup water
- 1 teabag of your preference.

Preparation:

1 Bring the water to a boil in a saucepan.
2 Add the lemon wedges to the water. Scoop out the pulp first and add it as well as the peels to the water for better blending. Simmer for 2 minutes.
3 Turn the heat off.
4 Add the vinegar, cayenne pepper and cinnamon powder to the mix. Stir.

5 Add the teabag. Let it steep. Remove.

6 Sip while warm.

Expert Advice:

For best results, make sure you have at least one cup every day. If you're taking only one helping of this tea per day, plan it for early in the morning. Let this tea be the first thing you have in the day. Make sure you put in a gap of at least 30 minutes between the tea and your breakfast. If you enjoy it and want to see more results, add a cup half an hour before lunch as well.

FAT LOSS TEA #3 – MINT MARVEL

This tea is fantastic for curbing hunger pangs and those random cravings that hit at odd hours during the day. The tea not only helps to detoxify the body and give it all sorts of nutrients, it also helps satiate hunger and leaves you feeling fuller for longer.

Ingredients:

- 1 tbsp. mint leaves- fresh, washed
- 1 teabag of your choice, preferably Green tea
- 1½ cups water
- ½ tsp. honey/ 1 small piece jaggery finely crushed

Preparation:

1 Add the water to a saucepan. Add the mint leaves.
2 Boil for 4-5 minutes. Watch for the water to take on a greenish hue. You should be able to smell the aroma of the mint leaves dissolving in the water. Wait until the mixture turns a more pronounced green.
3 Switch the heat off.
4 Add the teabag.
5 Let the brew steep for a few minutes- until the tea has infused with the mint mix nicely.
6 Remove the teabag.
7 Mix in the honey/ jaggery for sweetness. Adjust to taste.

Expert Advice:

You can take this particular tea with milk if you so desire, but for fast weight loss and maximum health benefits it is recommended that you do not. Take the tea after a meal (can be taken post lunch, but preferably time it for after dinner) because it improves the digestion process and helps the body settle quickly after a meal. It also prevents the munchies from striking late into the night!

Take these three tea brews as prescribed every day for 15 days and watch as the extra pounds all but fly off your body. Remember, for even more weight loss and giving your body some much needed strength you can work in the recipes we've discussed in the previous chapter as well.

CONCLUSION

Here's hoping that this e-book has opened your eyes up to a whole new lifestyle and given you a fitness option that's actually doable.

Who would've thought that's such a small change in your daily routine could bring about such a big difference in your health and life. When you take a moment to really think about it, adding tea to your daily diet is hardly something that's going to put you at an inconvenience. It's the least you can do for your health, but the results are nothing short of miraculous.

Remember, tea isn't supposed to be a substitute for other meals and foods in your diet. It's also not meant to replace an exercise program. There are no shortcuts to good health. What the tea cleanse aims to do is to help you kick start a new lifestyle.

To be able to continue losing weight even after you are done with the tea cleanse, it is recommended that you adopt a healthy lifestyle and focus on a nutritious, well-balanced diet and regular exercise. Adding these things to your lifestyle will only help augment the benefits of the tea cleanse.

Hopefully, when you see the amazing changes to your body at the end of the tea cleanse it is going to motivate you to push further and achieve more!

Sometimes it is just about finding the drive to do the things you anyway want to be able to do.

It's understandable that you want to see results, and this e-book guide is going to help you do just that.

Remember, tea, just like everything else, is an element of your lifestyle. You're going to have to work on the bigger picture and the smaller details to get the results you're looking for.

If you find it useful, do recommend it to friends and family. A happier, healthier environment and social circle are just a few clicks away!

PART 2

INTRODUCTION

Have you been feeling a little sluggish lately? Maybe you have found yourself being short tempered with those around you, or are too exhausted to do certain activities? When you cannot figure out what is happening in your external environment that affects your well-being, then it is highly likely that whatever you are dealing with is starting from inside of you. This is when you should try to detox, in order to restore yourself back to optimum health.

There are many different ways that you can choose to detox. Some include going on restrictive diets that will limit the types and amounts of foods that you can consume. Others require you to take in certain medicines or drugs in order to flush things out of your system. Choosing one of these options could leave you miserable as you try and cope with unpleasant side effects and question whether it was all worth it.

Instead, you can opt for a natural and gentle way to detox your system through the ultimate 10-day tea cleanse diet plan. Instead of keeping you hungry, going to extreme, or ingesting dangerous chemicals, this is a plan that helps you make healthy eating choices, while introducing powerful anti-oxidant tea into your system to help you cleanse all the dangerous toxins from your body.

You will find that this plan is pleasant and sustainable, while producing real results that will last you for a long period of time. In this book, are details on why this plan is important, the nutritional benefits that you can look forward to, and the results that you will get once you are done. Improve your health and well-being by trying out an effective diet plan that is purely results oriented. Read on for the ultimate tea cleanse.

Chapter 1: Everything You Need To Know About The Tea Cleanse

You would be amazed at the amount of toxins that are in your body at any given moment. Even though you are not purposely trying to ingest foods that will cause you damage, inevitably, you will. The problem with toxins is that they build up within you over time, and slowly but surely, begin to affect different parts of your body and your health.

Where exactly are these toxins coming from? Look at the basics. To begin with, the air that you breathe is likely filled with impurities from air pollution caused by dangerous gases being emitted by motor vehicles.

The water that you drink needs to be treated with chemicals in order for it to be safe for consumption, yet the same process that is meant to make it safe, also adds to its toxicity. If you eat vegetables that are not organic, you are filling your body with toxins, and the same counts for meat and anything else that you eat. Add to that all the processed food in the market and it is no wonder that your body is full of toxins.

It is possible to reduce the amount of toxins in our body in order to improve your overall health. One fantastic method is by detoxing the body, which simply means consuming something that will get rid of the toxins that are in your system. You will know that they are gone from the way that you will feel – cleaner, more energized and happier.

Without the right knowledge, it is unlikely that you will take the time needed to detox your body and get rid of all the dangerous items within you. Detoxing does not need you to take medicines or other substances that could cause damage to your health. Simply choosing an excellent ingredient, tea, can lead to a detox with great results.

A tea cleanse is essentially a short term plan, where you alter your existing diet including tea in specific ways so that you can cleanse your body of toxins that may be affecting your health.

It includes consumption of tea in addition to regular meals, and the elimination of foods that are termed as having danger elements or toxins from the diet. It also requires the elimination of exogenous toxins as much as possible to help the body operate at its optimum levels.

The reason that tea cleansing is an excellent option for detoxing the body is because it is a natural and gentle way to achieve great results.

You are not introducing harmful products into your body, neither are you limiting yourself to a liquid diet when you try a tea cleanse. Instead, you are using an ingredient with lots of anti-oxidants, and the capability of boosting overall health to get rid of the junk that is clogging up your system.

It is recommended that you carry out a tea cleanse at least once every six months if you eat an excellent healthy and balanced diet, or to have one every four months if your diet tends to be more unhealthy, meaning you do not drink enough water, or have at least 5 servings of fruit and vegetables each day.

CHAPTER 2: CHOOSING THE RIGHT TEA TO BENEFIT YOUR BODY

There are many different types of tea available on the market. These include black tea, white tea, flavored tea, herbal tea, green tea and more. For the purposes of detoxing, you need to focus on green tea.

Asian cultures have consistently consumed this tea, normally after meals and throughout the whole day. This is because green tea has excellent properties, since it is packed with anti-oxidants and vitamins. These are the benefits that you can expect from consuming green tea on a regular basis: -

- Builds up your immunity – Next time you have a cold or flu, instead of trying all sorts of over the counter medication that will leave your drowsy and without energy, try some green tea. It has properties that will fight those viruses safely, and you will feel much better in a short period of time. In addition to helping with these viruses, green tea also has medicinal value and can help your body to fight against arthritis, Alzheimer's, some cancers and even diabetes.

- Prevents dehydration – Green tea is able to prevent and cure dehydration.
- Weight Loss – There are anti-oxidants within green tea that help you to lose weight. This is because it is able to accelerate your metabolism, which leads to the body being able to burn energy. The great thing about this tea is that even when you are resting or sedentary, your body continues to burn up energy.

There are numerous varieties of green tea in the market, including flavored green tea, organic green tea, Asian green tea and so on. For the best results for a cleanse, consume the purest form of green tea that you can find, and avoid those which have additional flavors. In addition, you do not need to add any honey or other additives to your tea. Drinking it in its plain and natural form or with Jasmine is best.

There is one variety of green tea that is known as a Super Green Tea because of its potency regarding nutritional attributes that can help build your body. This is Matcha Tea from Japan. This is the best tea that you can use for a detox since it is ten times stronger than regular green tea. If it is not available, then you can make a choice from the following green teas: -

- Sencha Tea. This is often available in leaves of a variety of colors from the top of the shoot. It may be powdery or in long strands. It is often steamed or infused to bring out the best flavor.
- Gyokuru. This is also a Japanese Green Tea that is dark green in color. It has a very intense flavor and is attributed to being of excellent quality. It is one of the most expensive green teas that you will find in the market.

In addition to these options, there are more varieties which are similar, with minor differences that affect their overall aroma and subtle flavor. As you will be mixing these green teas with a range of ingredients in order to take advantage of the antioxidant properties, you may not feel that the actual flavor accounts for much, However, it is still worth noting which are the best, with the most effective properties so that you can bring out the best results from your cleanse.

It is possible that you will find these teas available locally at your supermarket or grocery store, however, it is advisable that you find the best varieties from natural food stores, as these are likely to be organic, which is recommended when you are attempting a detoxification tea cleanse.

THE ANTI-OXIDANT PROPERTIES OF GREEN TEA

As has been mentioned, there are numerous anti-oxidants and positive properties that you can find in green tea. These include the following: -

- Flavonoids – This includes a large category of antioxidants which include thearubigins, catechins and apicatechins.
- Polyphenols – These actually block the amount of damage one does to their DNA as a result of smoking tobacco or inhaling other chemicals that are toxic. The most important polyphenol that you will find in green tea is known as epigallocatechin gallate (EGCG). It is highly potent as an antioxidant, and is able to help with neurological disorders in the body, as well as with cardiovascular problems.
- Gallic Acid and Ascorbic Acid
- Minerals including chromium, selenium, manganese, zinc and phytochemical compounds.

So what do these anti-oxidant properties mean for the body? To being with, the properties in green tea are able to slow down the process of free radical release into the body, in addition, they prevent damage to DNA results. They are also more potent in their antioxidants than what you will find in certain vegetables such as spinach and garlic. It has also been proven to be much better for you than all the other different teas that you will find in the market.

They also are able to help prolong your life by building up your cells and preventing their damage. With close to ten times more antioxidants than fruits and vegetables, it is clear why green tea can be categorized as a super food.

Chapter 3: The Green Tea Cleanse And Your Internal Organs

The body is a fantastic instrument, which has been created to regenerate and cleanse itself so that it can function well. Unfortunately, we are giving the body much more than it can handle, and its natural cleansing ability is not enough to ensure that everything is in the right working order.

It is therefore necessary to detox, as well as to cleanse your essential organs for your body to work as expected. When done right, instead of shocking your system, you will create results that can last for the long run. That is why a tea cleanse is an excellent and effective options for detoxing the body.

Once you have chosen the right tea, it is necessary to understand exactly what it shall be doing within your body. Your body has five essential organs that need to be fully operational in order for you to enjoy optimum health. These organs, and the effect that green tea has on them, are described as follows: -

LIVER

Your liver is perhaps the most important organ in your body, as everything needs to go through it before it is filtered to other places. This means that you need that it is most likely to suffer from being packed full of toxins, and when this happens, it cannot function well and the entire body suffers. A green tea cleanse is a perfect solution for the restoration of your livers health. It helps the body to slowly get rid of toxins which have been accumulating and also with the elimination of waste that has been causing havoc within one's system.

LUNGS

Your lungs are used to take in air from the atmosphere and ensure that the right properties are made available for the rest of the body. This means that they act as a filter, getting rid of things that are in fumes, mold in the air, allergens and toxins that are floating around. When they are packed full of toxins, they cannot operate at their optimum levels, and the result is that you cannot take in proper deep breaths. Your breathing becomes shallow, and your lungs lose their power. This also means that your body will not receive the amount of oxygen that it needs. When you do a tea cleanse, you are filling your body with anti-oxidants, which in turn help to improve circulation in the capillaries within the lungs. In addition, the toxins within the lungs are diluted, and they are able to drain out which build up the strength of these organs.

SKIN

As you go through this tea cleanse, you will find that you are encouraged to exercise each day, so that you can rid your body of toxins through sweat. Your skin is essentially the largest organ that your body has, and therefore should be optimized when it comes to getting rid of toxins. Every time that you sweat, your skin excretes toxins that are building up below it, which improves its overall health, and also benefits your immune responses. The consumption of additional liquid and green tea help to make this process much easier.

BOWELS

Your bowels contain your intestinal tracts, which can hold an incredible amount of toxins that affect your health. You need to be able to clear these thoroughly. With this 10-day tea cleanse, you will go through a daily colon cleanse that shall help you to achieve this. This colon cleanse will eliminated secretions from all over the body that are stuck within your digestive tract, making your digestive system work more effectively. This will also lower the amount of dangerous toxins that are absorbed within your body, preventing constipation and improving colon functionality.

KIDNEYS

Your kidneys essentially help to flush out toxins through your urine, but, when they are busy fighting a barrage of toxins on their own, then this can be quite difficult to achieve. The color of your urine will alert you to the level of toxicity that you have in your body. With the green tea cleanse, you improve your overall hydration, which in turn helps your kidneys function much better. The properties from ingredients in this diet will also help to stimulate your bladder and within a short period of time, your urine will be an optimum color. The hidden added benefit of this is that you will begin to look and feel much slimmer that you did before, simply because you are well hydrated.

Chapter 4: The 10-Day Tea Cleanse Diet Plan

Within the next ten days, you would have completely transformed what is happening within your body, and will feel like you have a new lease of life following your tea cleanse diet. Your plan shall consist of two sections. There is what you must do in the morning in order to detox, and what must be done in the evening. In the morning, the focus is on replenishing the body of all the nutrients that it had lost during the night, particularly electrolytes. In the evening, the objective is to activate a colon cleanse to help clear the system.

GETTING STARTED

Before you begin this plan, you need to ensure that you have several things in place. To begin with, you must stock up with the following ingredients

- Green Tea, preferably Japanese Matcha Green Tea
- Fresh Lemons (At least 2 for each day)
- Fresh Ginger (At least one inch for each day)
- Senna Leaf
- Organic Acai Berry Juice
- Organic Barley Grass
- Organic Ginseng Powder
- Organic Lemon Grass
- Orange Peel
- Organic Liquorice Roots
- Organic Dandelion
- Organic Nettle Leaf

Tea is an excellent ingredient, but it is not enough on its own to guarantee that you get the best results. That is why you will find it is essential to combine it with some other ingredients. You need to use organic ingredients to prevent adding even more toxins into your body as a result of the cleanse. For the period of this week, the only drinks that you will consume are green tea and water.

In addition, for the entire week that you are doing this cleanse, you should ensure that you are free from social engagements, especially in the evenings. This is because you will be cleansing your colon, which will require you to be close to the bathroom through the evening.

MORNING CLEANSE

Before you start your morning cleanse each day, you need to prepare your body adequately. The moment that you get up, before you begin any of your daily activities, drink some warm to hot water in a 300 ml glass, that contains 3 tablespoons of fresh lemon juice and 1 teaspoon of fresh ginger (grated). This drink is able to accelerate your metabolism before you take start your day. 30 minutes after you have taken it in, you can drink your green tea morning cleanse.

The morning cleanse will consist of green tea, combined with other ingredients that have anti-oxidant properties and are categorized as super teas. These will help to activate your entire body and kick start the detox process each day. Follow this plan.

Day 1-2 – Green Tea with Acai Berry

Day 3 -4 – Green Tea with Barley Grass

Day 5-6 – Green Tea with Lemon Juice

Day 7 -8 – Green Tea with Ginseng

Day 9 – 10 – Green Tea with Ginger

After you have taken your morning cleanse, you need to continue drinking green tea throughout the day. Every one and a half hours, you should have a large cup of drink tea, without added sugar, honey or other ingredient. Presuming that you begin your day at 8.00 am and finish your day by 8.00 pm, this means you would have consumed 6-7 cups of green tea through the day, aside from your morning and evening cleanse.

Your morning cleanse shall be followed with a smoothie as your meal for breakfast. Recipes for your daily smoothies can be found in the following chapter. You can choose to try a new one each day, or to drink the same one for the period of your cleanse. They all have amazing detoxification and cleansing effects.

EVENING CLEANSE

To stimulate a colon cleanse, you need to include something with laxative properties into your tea. The colon cleanse, though not pleasant, is an excellent way to rig the body of toxins that have built up in the system. A natural and key element of your evening tea is Senna Leaf. Just like the morning cleanse, there are additional ingredients that can help to make a significant difference. Follow this plan.

Day 1-2 – Green Tea with Senna leaf and Lemon Grass

Day 3 -4 – Green Tea with Senna Leaf and Orange Peel

Day 5-6 – Green Tea with Senna Leaf and Liquorice Root

Day 7 -8 – Green Tea with Senna Leaf and Dandelion

Day 9 – 10 – Green Tea with Senna Leaf and Nettle Leaf

DAILY MEALS

With the morning and evening tea cleanses in place, you also need to ensure that any food you consume will help the entire process of cleansing and detoxing. This is now a plan that is designed to keep you hungry and miserable as you attempt to get your body into its best possible condition, instead, it is meant to help you feel better for longer in a short period of time.

You can be flexible in the meals that you eat, though you must follow these rules: -

- You need to have something to eat every six hours. This means that you will eat three times a day and will not have any snacks in between.
- You are permitted to eat non-starchy vegetables in whatever amounts you can handle for your meals. These include artichokes, tomatoes, kidney beans,

onions, bell peppers, Brussel sprouts, lettuce, cabbage, cauliflower, bean sprouts and so on.

- The best option you could choose is to eat all your vegetables raw. You could also choose to boil all of your vegetables and eat them as a clear broth (do not blend to make a soup). If you find this too difficult, you can grill or lightly fry them using extra virgin olive oil or coconut oil.
- You can season your food with fresh herbs, dried spices and salt and pepper. Other seasoning or flavors including ketchup and mayonnaise are not permitted.
- Every meal that you have must be accompanied with some protein. The proteins that you are allows include chicken, salmon, turkey, sardines, tofu and eggs. The portion of protein is also important, and should not exceed 150 gm per serving.
- You will not consume any carbohydrates during this cleanse, with exception of some fruit in your smoothies. This means that potatoes, meals with flour or wheat products, sugar and so on will not be consumed.
- During your tea cleansing period, you should not consume any processed foods or foods that have been deep fried as these will affect the results that you can achieve.
- You should not consume any alcohol during the period of the cleanse. If possible, also keep away from smoking cigarettes and consuming coffee as

well. Dairy products should be kept to the bare minimum of ½ cup of Greek Yoghurt each day.

OTHER ESSENTIAL TIPS

With your meals and your cleanses in check, here are some tips that will help you achieve the best possible results with minimal effort.

- Take some time to exercise. Detoxing and cleansing is all about clearing your body of toxins, and as you do so, you also elevate the rate at which your organs are able to operate. If you are sedentary, then most of your efforts will go to waste. It is almost like going to a birthday party knowing that at the end there will be cake. You wait for this in anticipation, and when there is no cake, you are sure to be disappointed. Therefore, for at least half an hour each day, get your body moving. You need to raise your heart rate, so a brisk walk or gentle jog will do the trick. In addition to increasing your blood flow and circulation, you will also sweat out some of those terrible toxins.
- Since you are likely to secrete more toxins through the skin due to exercise and taking in more fluids, you should ensure that your skin is able to work to your advantage. Skin brushing is an excellent way to improve the benefits you can get from this green

tea cleanse. All that is required is for you to brush your skin, moving towards your heart, to dislodge and remove all your dead skin cells. This will stimulate your lymph nodes which will in turn help to flush your body of dangerous toxins.

- Your mind and your body are interlinked, and one cannot be operating well if the other is not stable. Therefore, at the start of your day, spend some time in mediation. Fifteen minutes each day is enough. While you meditate, be sure to take in deep breaths through your nose, and breath out slowly through your mouth. You need to feel your abdomen rising and falling as you do this.

- There are sometime when it is not recommended that you detox, even when it is a light and natural detox like this one. If you are pregnant or breastfeeding, have certain health conditions such as high blood pressure, then you should not do this detox. If you are underweight, take the time to consult with your doctor before starting this detox and only move forward following their positive recommendation.

CHAPTER 5: DELICIOUS TEA RECIPES

For the most part, you can simply brew your green tea by steeping a green tea bag in hot water for three to four minutes and then drinking. Nonetheless, the way that you prepare your green tea will also depend on the type of green tea that you are using. Here are some tips to help you create the perfect cup.

JAPANESE MATCHA GREEN TEA

To prepare this tea, take one heaped teaspoon of powdered Japanese Matcha tea and stir into a cup of hot water. If possible, use a bamboo whisk, or stir very quickly. Once it is well mixed through, you can serve. There is no need to strain this tea. Drink it as is.

SENCHA GREEN TEA

This type of green tea is best infused. Take a large tea pot and fill it with hot water. Place within this tea pot at least two teaspoons of tea leaves, although you may prefer a little more for a stronger cup. The water temperature should be at a maximum of 90° C. The tea should be between yellow green and a dark green when ready which will be after around one to two minutes.

GYOKURU GREEN TEA

This green tea needs to be infused to bring out the best flavor. In a large tea pot, place one level tablespoon. Fill the tea pot with water at around 60° C. This is a relatively strong tea so you may need to take in smaller quantities. It should be left to infuse for at least 2 and a half minutes before drinking.

There are several things that you should keep in mind while brewing your green tea. TO begin with, you must use the right type of water for the best flavor. This means that you will avoid hard water or tap water, and instead opt for soft water. Soft water includes bottled mineral water which is devoid of toxins or too many foreign metals and chemicals. In addition, it will not contain chlorine which changes the delicate flavor of green tea.

However, you may want to experience all the benefits of green tea, while also amplifying the flavor of this super ingredient using other ingredients. The recipes in this section are ideal for you to try out as smoothies which you can take with your breakfast. Should you love the flavor of one (or all of them), you can choose to consume them during the day as well. Not only are they ideal for the detoxing period, they could also be incorporated into your everyday life after that to guarantee optimal health and well-being.

Remember, that every time you want to drink a cup of tea, you should brew, infuse or steep a fresh one. This will bring out the best attributes of the tea, and also help with the flavor.

GREEN TEA SMOOTHIE RECIPES

PINEAPPLE AND PEAR PARADISE GREEN TEA SMOOTHIE

Ingredients

300 ml Green Tea, chilled

½ cup peeled, cored and sliced Pineapple

½ peeled, cored and chopped Pear

Method

Place all the ingredients into a blender and blitz until there are no more chunks. Keep blitzing until it forms a thick juice. If it is a little too thick for your liking, add some more green tea. It should be smooth enough that you do not need to pass this through a strainer.

ISLAND DELICIOUS GREEN TEA SMOOTHIE

Ingredients

1 heaped teaspoon Green Tea Matcha Powder

1 Banana

½ Papaya, peeled and cut into cubes

½ Mango, peeled and cut into cubes

300 ml Coconut Milk

Method

In a blender, place all the ingredients and blend thoroughly. The final smoothie should be creamy and delicious. If you need to make it a little thinner, you can add in some soft water to the mix. Ensure that you always use the freshest of fruits for the best results. This recipe will not work as well with frozen fruit.

CREAMY GREEN TEA SMOOTHIE

Ingredients

300 ml Green Tea, chilled

½ Green Apple

½ cup Chopped Kale

2 tablespoons Greek Yoghurt

Method

Place all the ingredients into a blender and blitz until smooth. Pour into a tall glass and if you want a chilled beverage, add a few ice cubes. You can garnish this with a few sprigs of mint, or a lemon slice.

Orange, Grape Fruit, Lemon, Banana And Green Tea Smoothie

Ingredients

300 ml Green Tea, Chilled

1 Orange, peeled and cut into segments

1 Grapefruit, peeled and cut into segments

1 Lemon, juiced

1 Banana

½ cup Greek Yoghurt

1 teaspoon raw honey

Method

In a large blender, place all the ingredients and blitz until smooth. Ensure that you have blended well until you have a smooth consistency. Serve with orange rinds as a garnish.

BURSTING BERRIES GREEN TEA SMOOTHIE

Ingredients

300 ml Green Tea, Chilled

1/3 cup Raspberries (fresh)

1/3 cup Blueberries (fresh)

¼ cup Greek Yoghurt

Method

Place all the ingredients into a large blender and blitz until very smooth and creamy. If you do not have any fresh berries, you can use frozen ones for a particularly chilled smoothie on a hot day.

CHAPTER 6: THE ADDED BENEFITS OF INGREDIENTS IN THIS PLAN

The ingredients that have been included as a part of this diet plan were not chosen at random. They all have benefits that extend the effectiveness of the green tea, while also ensuring that your body gets everything that it needs to remain healthy. This section explains what these additional ingredients contain.

KALE

In addition to being a rich source of Vitamin K which is not found in many other ingredients, kale is also full of phytonutrients.

GINSENG

There are a total of eleven different plant varieties that are given the name ginseng, ant they are all herbs where the root is used. They are able to increase overall energy, as well as help with controlling blood sugar. It also has anti-inflammatory effects that are useful when detoxing, and the added benefit of improving cognitive function which helps with clear thinking.

PINEAPPLES

This fruit is an excellent source of Vitamin C. This is a vitamin that acts as an antioxidant wants it has been introduced to the body. When combined with green tea, you are sure that your immune system gets a significant boost and has added protection.

BARLEY GRASS

This is excellent for maintaining fantastic skin, and also for the regeneration of cells and tissues that have bene damaged. It also is able to balance the body in regards to acids and alkaline, which can help when purging the body of toxins. Like other ingredients included in this cleanse, barley grass also contains a considerable amount of anti-oxidant properties. You can use it to fight addictions, which can help with your continued health after you complete the cleanse.

KIDNEY BEANS

Their shape and the organ that they benefit in this cleanse are interlinked, and you can expect that kidney beans will benefit the kidney.

APPLES

On this plan, you are not permitted any sugar in your tea, as it has been processed to be in its current form. Apples add sweetness to your smoothies, in addition to being packed with nutrients.

PEARS

This ingredient is rich in fiber, which helps when you need to carry things through and clear your colon. It also has a fantastic flavor.

Citrus Fruits

These include oranges, lemons and grapefruits, and they have a large number of detoxifying attributes that make them suitable for use with this cleanse. Lemon juice has long been used for detoxification within the body, as well as boosting the metabolic system. Citrus fruits also include a lot of Vitamin C, as well as flavonoids. Other minerals which help to boost the body's functionality include magnesium, potassium, iron and phosphorus.

GREEK YOGHURT

Consuming dairy is not recommended while on this diet, however, Greek Yoghurt is allowed. You only need a small quantity to get excellent smoothness to drinks, and it is packed full of protein which is required at each meal. It also tastes delicious.

ACAI BERRIES

Blueberries have long been attributed with having antioxidant properties, yet, they do not come close to what the acai berry has to offer. This berry that is found within the Amazon rainforest is packed full of anti-oxidants, and it is able to boost overall energy, as well as build up the immune system. When detoxing with green tea, it helps to improve the health of the cells in the body as well as to aid in overall digestion. This is because it is also a rich source of fiber.

ARTICHOKES

Although it is recommended that you should eat your vegetables raw, you would need to boil your artichokes while on this plan. They have the added advantage of being delicious and the best foods that you can give your liver when cleansing. They help with metabolic function, and are known for their properties of detoxification.

CHAPTER 7: THE BASICS OF THE ANTI-INFLAMMATORY DIET

The word 'diet' is seen as a dirty word by some, as it denotes struggling to eat meals that you do not enjoy in a bid to reach a specific target so that you can improve your overall body image. Diet actually refers to the types of food that one eats, which means it is more descriptive than descriptive.

Based on the initial understanding of the word, the Anti-Inflammatory diet that has been created by Dr. Andrew Weil is not actually a diet that leads to weigh loss. It is more a plan of eating that can be sustained over a long period to ensure one reaches their optimum health.

Inflammation is not actually negative, as it helps the body receive extra nourishment and improves immune activity when a certain area has been injured or infected. It is an automatic response. This response has a powerful effect on the whole body, which then affects general wellbeing.

Inflammation is not caused by bacteria or viruses such as you can expect from infection, it simple is the way the body chooses to handle it. It goes through various stages, the first in being the area becoming irritated. After this occurs, the site where the infection is then going through suppuration, a process in which pus is discharged to aid in healing of the wounded area.

There are two more types of inflammation, and these are referred to as acute inflammation and chronic inflammation. Acute information happens in the short term, advancing relatively fast and becoming quite severe. Chronic inflammation takes a longer term approach, sometimes, even being in the body for years on end. The longer we have inflammation, the worse off our bodies are, and that is why chronic inflammation is responsible for various diseases. This type of inflammation does not allow the tissues to heal properly. To determine whether you have inflammation, you need to check for the following symptoms; heat, pain, swelling, redness and injured function.

Chronic inflammation which occurs when inflammation persists for a long period, or when someone is highly stressed, out of shape or exposed to toxins can result in significant, and sometimes even life threatening conditions. The most common ones include cancers, obesity, heart disease, rheumatoid arthritis and Alzheimer's. When one suffers from chronic inflammation, taking a range of medications can help to minimize the symptoms, but changing one's approach to food can ultimately eliminate the root cause of the problem. This means that this diet is more natural and sustainable, then a myriad of medicines that you may buy off the counter.

ESSENTIAL RULES

The Anti-Inflammatory diet is not about being restrictive with your meals, rather it calls for you to be able to adapt. Therefore, you need to keep the following rules in mind.

- Focus on eating fresh foods, and cut down on junk or fast food, as well as processed foods.
- Aim for the average calorie intake required by men and women, which is 2000 and 3000 calories respectively each day.
- Ensure that you keep an excellent mix of nutrients, the best being 40% carbohydrates, 30% of fat and 30% of protein at each meal.
- Elevate the flavors of your meals with spices like ginger and turmeric, as these are known to have anti-inflammatory effects.
- Watch how you cook, and choose methods that retain the nutrients inside your food. Grilling, baking and steaming are excellent options, whereas frying should not be used for food preparation.

Benefits Of The Anti-Inflammatory Diet

When there is something that is wrong within your body, most often there is some inflammation. To communicate this to your brain, a signal of pain is sent and the discomfort will have you seeking some remedy. To prevent continuous and consistent pain, it is best to try an anti-inflammatory diet. The immediate effect that this will have is to reduce the amount of inflammation, and this will then reduce the pain that you are experiencing.

Another benefit is what this diet inside your body to reduce inflammation. People with chronic illnesses begin to feel the benefits of this diet after several weeks. Take for example a cancer patient, who is looking for some form of natural treatment to boost their chemotherapy or radiation results. The foods that are in this diet are excellent for maintaining health, reducing inflammation and in creating an alkaline environment. Cancer cells thrive in an acidic environment, and will die in an environment that does not encourage their growth.

Elements of this diet, including the intake of flax seeds, drinking large amounts of water and drink tea, and preparing meals that do not contain processed foods or junk. The pure foods that you eat go into your body and help to stabilize it, for example, the flax seed going to the liver and helping to repair it. Juicing vegetables also fills the body with necessary anti-oxidants.

All these benefits are amazing, but if you have never thought that inflammation could affect you, you might question why you even need to explore an anti-inflammatory diet. This is especially true if you are not suffering from a chronic illness, experience close to no pain at all, and are generally in good health. To begin with, everyone suffers from inflammation, and the older you get, the more it becomes. When you are healthy, it becomes more challenging to see the symptoms on the outside that reflect what is happening to you on the inside. There is inflammation that you can see on the outside, such as a swelling when you have an injury. It is a little trickier to establish where within your body you have inflammation.

The reason that you need this diet, even if you question whether you have issues, is because it calls for a change in your lifestyle which ensures that you minimize your chances of complications as a result of inflammation. It is the first step to taking control of your overall health, maintaining a good body weight and preventing health scares and diseases. Prevention is so much better than cure, and that is why when you get into a car to go on a journey, you put on your seatbelt. You know that in case of a crash, it will prevent you from experiencing too much injury.

CHAPTER 8: CONDITIONS THAT CAN BE TREATED BY THE ANTI-INFLAMMATORY DIET

There are several illnesses that benefit directly from an anti-inflammatory diet. When this diet is made a way of life, patients experience less pain than ever and find that other symptoms they were experiencing also reduce.

Although the anti-inflammatory diet is primarily meant to treat diseases that occur as a result of chronic inflammation, it can also help with conditions that are caused by acute inflammation. This is especially true if these conditions last for several weeks. Some of these include the following:

- Acute tonsillitis
- Acute bronchitis
- Acute dermatitis
- Acute sinusitis
- Acute meningitis
- Acute appendicitis

Some medical practitioners claim that this type of diet is excellent for the 'itis' diseases, which is all the conditions that end with the letters itis.

The anti-inflammatory diet is most effective when it is used to help with conditions from chronic inflammation. Here are some of these illnesses.

Rheumatoid Arthritis

This is an illness that is primarily caused by inflammation, and it can affect anyone, no matter what age they may be. What happens is that the immune system launches an attack which affects the bones. In the morning, a patient will experience stiffness and pain in their joints, and these joints can also become swollen and feel tender to the touch. Although this condition cannot be cured, the symptoms can be managed. Most people will opt for medication which has side effects that are unpleasant. An anti-inflammation diet contains Omega 3 acids, which help to reduce these symptoms substantially and safely.

To get better, delicious curries that have plenty of ginger can make a difference within a few weeks. Furthermore, this diet is rich in omega 3 acids, antioxidants, fiber and flavonoids, which all work together to minimize inflammation.

Osteoarthritis

As you become older, your joints will begin to natural wear down which is a condition that is known as osteoarthritis. This condition is incredibly painful, and can limit a person's movement significantly. By consuming foods as in the anti-inflammatory diet, it is possible to get help and reduce all that pain. In essence, this chronic condition can then be managed.

PSORIASIS

This is a skin condition that has no cure. A person will have 'outbreaks' where parts of their skin (on any place in the body) become inflamed and in some cases, this can even become painful. This diet can help with the management of symptoms such that the person being affected may not even believe that they have any disease at all.

OTHER CONDITIONS

The anti-inflammatory diet is able to treat and manage several other conditions. These include hypertension, as it can help to lower a person's blood pressure. It is also helpful for conditions that are chronic, such as strokes and cancers. Heart disease can be reduced as well. Then there is the benefit of managing obesity, as the subsequent weight loss from eating well can help reduce the pressure that is placed on the joints.

CHAPTER 9: ESSENTIAL FOODS OF THE ANTI-INFLAMMATORY DIET

The best way to ensure that you have the best mix of ingredients is to use the Anti-Inflammatory Food Pyramid. It contains the following: -

- At the base of the pyramid is water, which you need to drink throughout the day. Most diets recommend at least eight glasses a day although it is better to consume more than this amount.
- Next, you should eat a healthy amount of vegetables (5 servings a day) and fruit (4 servings a day), preferably in their raw form.
- Following this and the next step up in the pyramid is whole and cracked grains (3 servings each day), whole meal pastas (3 times in a week) and beans and legumes (once a day).
- This if followed by healthy fats at around 5 servings each day, which includes delicious fruits like avocado and extra virgin olive oil
- At least two to six times in a week, you should consume some fish and seafood.
- For protein, try at least one serving of whole soy foods each day. This is followed by other sources of protein, such as eggs and cheese which you need to consume at least twice a week. Also included here are lean meats as well as skinned poultry.

- Three steps from the top of the pyramid is healthy herbs and spices, which include garlic. You can have these in unlimited amounts so make sure to use them to elevate your meals
- You can also eat an unlimited amount of Asian mushrooms which are credited with having anti-ageing qualities in addition to anti-inflammatory ones.
- The next step up includes dietary supplements which you can take in on a daily basis. These also include teas such as green and white tea. Having two to four cups of tea each day is recommended.
- Just before the top is red wine, and you can have one glass of red wine each day.
- At the very top of this pyramid are your healthy sweets, such as dark chocolate. Save these for special occasions as you can only eat them sparingly.

YOUR BALANCED DIET

The following is an estimation of how you can balance your meals if you are on a diet where you take in 2,000 calories a day for women and 3,000 calories a day for men. Women should consume 180 grams of carbs, 60 grams of fat and 100 grams of protein on a daily basis. Men require 270 grams of carbs, 80 grams of fat and 120 grams of protein on a daily basis. Both men and women should consume 40 grams of fiber each day.

These numbers are averaged and can go up or down by 10%.

The foods that you choose to consume should have a low glycemic load. In addition, if you stick to the pyramid, you will be filling your body up with anti-inflammatory substances which include antioxidants from fruits and vegetables, high amounts of fiber, essential nutrients such as magnesium, anti-inflammatories, oleocanthal, omega 3s and isoflavones.

FOODS TO MINIMIZE

It would be close to impossible to avoid certain foods, especially if you have been eating them for years, but, it is possible to minimize certain items. This is because there are some foods which are known to cause inflammation in the body, and reducing their intake will lead to significant relief. For the best results, you need to cut down on flour made from wheat and all the products that are made from wheat, sugar, and processed snacks that have been packaged. Wheat contains gluten which for many people causes inflammation. If you must eat anything that is processed, avoid packaged products which include high fructose corn syrup.

When it comes to fatty foods, you need to eat more foods with monounsaturated fats than those with saturated and polyunsaturated fats. This will mean that foods such as butter and cream should be reduced. Fats which have been processed such as vegetable shortening and margarine should be minimized almost completely. They can be replaced with nut butter, and mashed avocado.

Not all protein is good for you, and you need to minimize the amount of animal protein that you consume. This means cutting down on red meat such as beef and lamb. If you feel that you must consume some red meat, make sure that it is organic. Meat that is not organic contains arachidonic acid, which has been found to cause inflammation. In addition, you will need to cut down on your intake of dairy products, especially milk.

There are some vegetables that you should avoid as they can result in inflammation. These include eggplants, potatoes and tomatoes. They substance solanine is present in these, although you are unlikely to find it in any other vegetables.

FOODS TO MAXIMIZE

A simple way to know which carbs to eat is simple to ask yourself, how brown is it? Give up your white rice and processed wheat and opt for bulgur wheat and brown rice. These are rich in fiber, and much better for your body.

When it comes to fats, consume more extra virgin olive oil as well as other organic oils including canola and sunflower oils. When selecting your oils, it is even better if they have been cold-pressed. You can also find excellent fats in fish, such as mackerel and salmon. These will have Omega 3 fatty acids as well, which can help control inflammation.

For proteins, you need to increase the amount of vegetable proteins you consume such as beans. In addition, you should increase the amount of fish and seafood that you consume. Should you take in any red meat, limit your intake to 400 gm a month for the best results. All your meat should be lean, and white meat like chicken and turkey should not include the skin.

The bulk of your meals will be made up of fruits and vegetables, and these need to be organic. For the best fruits, you need to try those that are in season and fresh. When choosing these fruits and vegetables, keep the colors of the rainbow in mind as you make your selections. These vegetables and fruits that have bright and rich colors, are often the ones that have the best nutrients.

Flavor will transform the joy you have when eating, and including spices is a sure way to amplify flavor. Turmeric is a spice that has recognized anti-inflammatory qualities, and you can also introduce rosemary as a herb.

If you have a habit of grabbing a snack at certain times of the day, as you do not have enough time to create an entire meal, choose snacks with anti-inflammatory qualities, such as pumpkin seeds, walnuts and flaxseeds.

There is an anti-inflammatory super food which has more antioxidants than any other food on this diet. That is tart-cherries, which you should try to consume as often as possible.

SUPPLEMENTS

When you study the layers that you need to go up with the anti-inflammatory diet, you will notice that near the top of the pyramid there is room for supplements. Your body needs to have a range of essential vitamins and minerals to get the best out of this diet. As you eat healthier, you will invest more of these, though taking a supplement is a sure way or preventing anything from going wrong. You need to have the following each day: -

- Vitamin E – 400 IU each day
- Vitamin C – 200 mg a day
- Vitamin D – as much as you can get from the sun
- Carotenoids – 10,000 IU each day

- Calcium – 700 mg a day
- Selenium – 200 micrograms

SPICES

You would have noted by now that turmeric is king when it comes to a spice with anti-inflammatory qualities. There are some other spices you can try which also have excellent effects.

Ginger, both fresh and ground is an excellent option. This is followed by cinnamon, which has a war flavor that is ideal for use on breakfast oats or curry dishes. Baking with cinnamon is also favored as it has a delicious aroma and also tastes very good.

Garlic is great for reducing inflammation, particularly in people who are suffering from hypertension. Having garlic within this diet helps to build flavor as well as reduce the symptoms from other conditions like arthritis.

Black pepper and cayenne pepper contain capsaicinoids, which have properties for anti-inflammation. They also help to elevate the flavors of foods. Cloves in any form are also great, and they can be added to stews and soups, as well as a range of baked goods.

Chapter 10: Your 5 Week Anti-Inflammatory Diet Plan

This is the moment that you take control of your life forever, by starting on this 5-week anti-inflammatory diet plan. This plan does not stop within five weeks, as the diet is intended to be a change in your lifestyle. However, you will find that within this period, you will have adjusted to all the changes that you have made in your diet, such that, it becomes a way of life. Here is a five-week plan that will guarantee you get the results that you need.

Week 1 – Getting On Track

The first day of this week shall be spent doing an assessment of your body and your expectations. You will need a sheet of paper where you can put down your vital statistics. These will include your weight and body measurements. Added to this will be information on how much sleep you get in general each night, what you would eat on a typical day, the amount of alcohol and coffee you consume, and whether you get any exercise. Illnesses that you currently have should be included here as well, in addition to any bad habits you have like smoking or taking drugs.

Following this physical assessment, you will do an emotional assessment to establish where you are mentally in regards to your feelings about yourself and the diet, and your hopes as to the end result. When you put this all down on paper, you will have an excellent idea of what motivates you, which is important if you want to see a real change in your life.

For the second day of this week, you will map a way forward. This will include certain changes that you may need to make. In your day, you need to factor in 30 minutes of exercise, eight hours of sleep each night and fixed meal times for three meals and two snacks.

Remember that your diet plan is not meant to be restrictive, instead, it will help you make better choices. Therefore, you can look at how to adjust what you are already eating to fit within this plan. If you find this a challenge, here is what you need to do for the rest of this week.

Start by increasing your fruit and vegetable intake. At breakfast, make sure the first thing that you eat is fruit, and if you are having anything else, incorporate fruit into this as well. For your snacks, make some fruit smoothies and if you need milk, use soya milk. For dessert at both lunch and dinner, ensure you have some fruit after meals.

In addition, eliminate all processed food from your diet, and focus on eating brown instead of white when it comes to your carbohydrates. Switch up carbonated drinks with green tea and water. Juice your vegetables if you find it a challenge to consume all the portions that are required in a day. The first week of this diet plan is the most challenging, but by the time the week draws to a close, you will begin to notice that you have less cravings than you did before, and that you have better control of your own eating habits than you through possible.

Here is a menu plan for Weeks 1 and 2.

	Day 1	Day 2	Day 3	Day 4	Day 5	Day 6	Day 7
Brea kfas t	Gree	Veg	Poach	Fruit	Coco	Fres	Poac
	n	e	ed	sal	n	h	he
	T	t	eg	ad	ut	f	d
	e	a	g	wi	a	r	eg
	a,	b	wi	th	n	u	g
	O	l	th	chi	d	it	wi
	at	e	W	a	C	w	th
	m	J	ho	se	h	it	W
	e	u	leg	ed	er	h	h
	al	ic	rai	s	ry	c	ol
	a	e	n		P	o	eg
	n	,	to		or	c	ra
	d	a	ast		ri	o	in
	B	n	,		d	n	to
	er	d	Ap		ge	u	as

	ries, One Banana	Sliced banana with cinnamon	ple			t and nuts.	t, Apple
Snack	Handful of Walnuts	Handful of Al l	Hummus and Carrot Sti	Green Tea and Strawberri	Blueberries and S	Oat muffin and d	Celery Sticks and Alm

91

		monds	cks, Green Tea	es	oya Yoghurt	Green Tea	ond Butter
Lunch	Grilled Salmon with Spinach Salad a	, vegetable lasagna	Vegetable Broth with Avocado Salad and vinaigrette, M	Grilled skinless chicken breast with mixed vegetabl	Green salad, Tofu and wholegrain wrap	Lemonand Herb Salad with s ar	Vegetable Broth with Avocado Salad and vina

	nd Olive oil/ Lemon dressing. Mango		ango	es and avocado. Wholegrain wrap.		dines, Apple	igrette, Mango
Snack	Green Tea, A	Hummus an	Watermelon Sm	Hummus, Avocad	Celery Sticks a	Banana Sm	Strawberry S

	vocado on Rye	dCelery, Green Tea	oothie	o, Rye Crackers	ndAlmond Butter	oothie	moothie
Dinner	Vegetarian Curry with Brow	Steamed Trout with Gi	Spaghetti and Turkey Meatballs, Ka	Vegetable Soup with an Orange	Shitake mushroom and grille	Bean burger, sweet p	Vegetarian Curry with Brown Ri

	nRice	nger, garlic and lime and butternut squa	le, Banana		d Salmon with quinoa and vegetables	otatoes, wholemeal bun and salad	ce

95

		s h					
Trea t	Glass of re d W in e		Dark Ch oc ol at e on e sq ua re		Glass of re d wi n e		Dark C h oc ol at e o ne sq ua re

WEEK 2 – MAKE A COMMITMENT

Using the guidance of meals from week 1, you should begin to understand where you can make substitutions and prepare your food differently. In this week, you can prepare your meals using the plan from week 1, though you will make some special considerations.

To begin with, you need to increase the amount of cruciferous vegetables that you consume. This will mean that you should eat more Brussel sprouts, kale and lettuces. In addition, make sure that you consume a considerable amount of turmeric and fresh ginger.

You can use these in smoothies, veggie juices or aromatic curries.

Hopefully, you have managed to get half an hour of exercise each day. Increase this to 45 minutes and include some yoga as well as something that is aerobic in nature. Ensure that you are not consuming any sugar with your meals, it does nothing for you nutritionally and can affect your efforts to minimize your inflammation.

WEEK 3 – DEALING WITH TEMPTATION

At this point, it is likely that you have managed to stay the course of the diet, and you see changes in your body and the way that you feel. Just when things seem to be going well, you will find that temptation begins to creep its ugly head in. You may tell yourself that you have made progress, so you can have just one cookie, or now you can choose something that would be a 'cheat' food, and it will do no permanent damage.

This is where you need to evaluate what you want to achieve at the end of your journey, and say no to things that will veer you of course. Also, ensure that you are still doing certain things right including getting enough sleep and exercise so that you can stay on course.

This week you can be flexible with your menu, keeping in mind that you need to grill your meats and ensure they are lean, as well as to eat fruit several times a day.

You will find that fruit smoothies are delicious and filling, so have some during the day. Bridge all your meals with green tea, and if you have this tea warm, it will be easier for you to sustain yourself between meals.

The type of training you do this week should be focused on resistance, to build up your muscles which can help to reduce your inflammation. Simple exercises like push-ups can have a fantastic effect.

Should you feel puckish at any time during the day, a handful or two of blueberries or raspberries will give your body and excellent dose of antioxidants.

WEEK 4 – WORK ON YOURSELF INSIDE OUT

With your meals under control, and your temptation taken care of, you need to review your general stress levels and mental wellbeing. Stress can cause you to leave your plan, or to experience inflammation even when you are making great strides to improve. Your stress will be elevated if you are not getting the right amount of sleep, or cutting back on your exercise. Before you begin to tackle the plan for this week, take some time to figure out what could be causing you stress and deal with it.

	Day 1	Day 2	Day 3	Day 4	Day 5	Day 6	Day 7

Breakfast	Green Tea, Oatmeal and Berries, One Banana	Millet porridge prepared with coconut milk. Blue	Poached egg with Wholegrain toast, Apple	Millet porridge prepared with coconut milk. Blueberries	Green Tea, Oatmeal and Berries, One Banana	Fresh fruit with coconut and nuts.	Quinoa with blueberries, handful of almonds

		berries					
Snack	Handful of Walnuts	Spicy Smoothie	Hummus and Carrot Sticks, Green Tea	Green Tea and Strawberries	Blueberries and Soya Yoghurt	Oat muffin and Green Tea	Celery Sticks and Almond Butter
Lunch	Grilled Salmo	Mexican salad,	Beet Salad with Gi	Grilled skinless ch	Salmon cakes	Lemon and H	Broccoli and Cranb

100

	n	dr	ng	ick	w	e	er
	w	es	er	en	it	r	ry
	it	si	an	br	h	b	Sa
	h	n	d	ea	vi	S	la
	S	g	Ca	st	n	a	d,
	pi	fr	rr	wi	ai	l	wi
	n	o	ot	th	gr	a	th
	a	m	s	mi	et	d	cri
	c	A		xe	te	w	sp
	h	v		d	a	i	ap
	S	o		ve	n	t	pl
	al	c		ge	d	h	es
	a	a		ta	la	s	
	d	d		bl	rg	a	
	a	o,		es	e	r	
	n	M		an	sa	d	
	d	a		d	la	i	
	O	n		av	d	n	
	li	g		oc		e	
	v	o		ad		s	
	e			o.		,	
	oi			W		A	
	l/			ho		p	
	L			le		p	
	e			gr		l	
	m			ai		e	
	o			n			
	n			wr			
	d			ap			

				.			
	ressing. Mango						
Snack	Green Tea, Avocadoon Rye	Pineapple smoothie with Ginger	Watermelon Smoothie	Hummus, Avocado, Rye Crackers	Ginger and Turmeric Smoothie	Banana Smoothie	Strawberry Smoothie
Din	Vege	Stea	Spag	Veget	Fried	Lent	Salm

ner	t a ri a n C u rr y w it h B r o w n Ri c e	m e d Tr o ut w it h Gi n g er , g ar lic a n d li m e a n d b ut te	he tti an d Tu rk ey M ea tb all s, Ka le, Ba na na	ab le So up wi th an Or an ge	e g g w it h gr e e n sa la d	il s c u r r y	o n ca ke s an d Br oc co li, B an an a

103

		rn ut s q u as h					
Trea t	Glas s o f r e d W in e		Dark Ch oc ol at e on e sq ua re		Glass of re d w in e		Dark C h oc ol at e o n e sq ua re

WEEK 5 – A LIFESTYLE CHANGE

This week, you can refer to the menu from week 4 for your meals. It is essential that you make some permanent changes if your intention is to enjoy a complete change in your lifestyle and a brilliant future.

To begin with, you need to remove any items in your home that could get you to slip off the wagon. These will include sugar, dairy products, processed foods, white carbohydrates and soft drinks. Replace these with Stevia, soya products, fresh fruits and vegetables, nuts, brown carbohydrates and lots of green tea. When you do not have the foods that do not serve your health around you, it is possible to make smarter choices.

Watch out for the excuses that will creep up on you to stop you from making these changes. These would include the effects your changes will have on your family, the fact that you do not want to crave what you love, or that you will do it later. This lifestyle change is transformative, and the benefits cannot be underestimated. Make the tough choices now, and look forward to a brighter and healthier future.

Chapter 11: Essential Recipes And Cooking Tips

Your Anti-Inflammatory meals can be especially delicious if you try out these recipes.

Breakfast

Oatmeal And Berries
Ingredients

1 cup oatmeal

2 large teaspoons of mixed berries (blueberries, raspberries, strawberries)

½ cup natural yoghurt

½ cup water

Method

In a medium pan, heat up the water and stir in the oatmeal. Allow to heat through and cook. Take off the heat and stir in the natural yoghurt until you are left with a thick, creamy consistency. Add in the mixed berries, transfer into a bowl, and enjoy. This is enough for two servings.

Coconut And Cherry Porridge

Ingredients

2 cups of oats

4 cups of coconut milk

3 large spoons of chia seeds

2 large spoons cocoa

½ cup coconut (grated or shavings)

½ cup cherries

Honey to taste

Stevia to taste

Garnish with grated chocolate

Method

Take a large pan and place it on medium heat. Place the oats, coconut milk. Chia seeds, cocoa and stevia in the pan. When the oats have come to a boil, you should reduce the heat to low and simmer for about five minutes.

Take off the heat and place into a large bowl. Top with the rest of the ingredients and serve. This can also make an excellent and warming snack on a cold day.

LUNCH

TUNA SALAD WITH CRUSTY BREAD

Ingredients

½ can of chunks Tuna in Brine or Olive Oil

½ cup butterhead lettuce leaves

¼ large white onion cut into rings

Several slices of cucumber

1 stick celery chopped into slices

1 mashed avocado mixed with juice of one lemon

2 slices 7 grain bread – lightly toasted.

Method

In a medium bowl, combine the drained tuna, white onion, cucumber and celery. Next, take the slices of bread and lay them out on a plate. On each slice, place several lettuce leaves. Top with the tuna mixture and place a dollop of the mashed avocado on the very top. Serve with a delicious smoothie for a filling meal.

BEET SALAD WITH CARROTS AND GINGER

Ingredients

1 cup beetroot raw, peel and grate

1 cup carrots, peel and grate

1 teaspoon ginger, fresh

½ cup apple juice

1 large spoon extra virgin olive oil

Sprinkling of salt

Method

In a medium bowl, place the carrots and the beetroot. Mix until well combined. In a separate bowl, create the dressing by mixing the ginger, apple juice, olive oil and salt. Once combined, pour this into the beetroot mixture and toss well. Serve.

DINNER

TURKEY MEATBALLS AND SPAGHETTI

Ingredients

200 grams whole-wheat Spaghetti

200 grams Turkey mince

½ cup chopped whole-wheat bread slices

½ red onion chopped into small pieces

1 egg

1 handful chopped Italian parsley

Salt and Pepper

1 stick butter

1 teaspoon fresh chopped chives

Dollop of cream

Method

In a large pot full of boiling hot water, bring the spaghetti to a boil until it is al-dente. While the spaghetti is boiling, take a bowl and in it, place the turkey mince, chopped bread, red onion, egg, parsley, salt and pepper. Mix well and roll into balls that are around one inch in diameter.

In a frying pan, melt the butter over medium heat, being careful not to allow it to brown. Gently fry all the meat balls until brown and cooked through. Take them out of the pan. Add the dollop of cream and the chives to the pan to create a sauce. If you want more sauce, add a little more cream. Toss the spaghetti in the sauce and serve.

BROCCOLI AND CRANBERRY SALAD WITH CRISP APPLES

Ingredients

2 cups fresh broccoli, cut into florets

¼ cup cranberries (dried)

2 fresh apples

¼ cup sunflower seeds

½ cup yoghurt (plain)

¼ red onion, chopped into small pieces

1 tablespoon Dijon mustard

Honey to taste

Method

In a large bowl, mix together the broccoli, sunflower seeds, cranberries, apples and onion. Ensure that they have combined well. In a separate bowl, create a dressing with yoghurt, honey and mustard. Mix the dressing together with the vegetables and serve. For better flavor, ensure that the salad is chilled.

SNACKS

CHOC AND NUTS

Ingredients

One large bar of dark chocolate

Two handfuls of walnuts

Method

Break the chocolate up into pieces and mix in a large sealable container. Take the walnuts and chop up into large pieces. Add to the chocolate and combine well. When you need a snack, eat one tablespoon of this mixture with a drink.

Smoothies

Spicy Smoothie

Ingredient

¼ cup blueberries

¼ cup pawpaw

1 large banana

1 large spoon chia seeds

¼ teaspoon cinnamon

¼ teaspoon turmeric

Dash of salt and cayenne pepper

¼ teaspoon ginger

1 teaspoon stevia

1 cup cold green tea

Method

Place all the ingredients in a blender and blitz well. If you feel that the smoothie is too thick you can thin it out with a little more green tea.

GINGER AND TURMERIC SMOOTHIE

Ingredients

1 cup almond milk (unsweetened)

½ cup peaches

1 large banana

½ teaspoon turmeric

½ teaspoon chia seeds

½ teaspoon cinnamon

½ teaspoon ginger

Honey to taste

Method

Take all the ingredients and place them in a blender. Ensure that all the items have been well blended until you reach a nice consistency.

Cooking Tips

- Wondering what you can do with beans? Beans are highly versatile and a delicious addition to many meals. Include beans in a soup or stew, and you will be amazed at how good they will taste, and the amount of nutrition that they add to the meal.

- A refreshing beverage that you can drink all through the day is green tea. It has excellent anti-inflammatory qualities in addition to being light in flavor.

- The type of meat that you choose and the way that you cook that meat is essential for the success of this plan. Avoid eating meat that has been fried or breaded, and instead opt for meats that have been grilled or baked. In addition, ensure that all the cuts that you choose are as lean as possible.

- When preparing your vegetables, steam them instead of boiling or frying them. Steam helps to retain the maximum number of units, and you will also end up with crisp vegetables that are ready to eat, instead of soggy and limp offerings.

- Take the time to evaluate what you normally eat, and then make certain adjustments. Learn to make more use of your oven and enjoy how great your food can taste when you use a barbecue.

- Juicing your vegetables and eating your fruits is a great way to ensure that you get the maximum number of servings a day. Adding in some spice helps elevate natural flavors and create signature drinks.
- As you prepare to cook your meal, check and see how many of the ingredients that you are using are organic. Try as much as possible to ensure that all of them are, as this will reduce the number of chemicals that you ingest into your body.

CHAPTER 12: TIPS TO MAKE IT LAST

You want to ensure that once you have completed the five weeks that are outlined within this plan, that you can continue for a lifetime. Here are some tips that are sure to ensure you make this positive life change.

DO NOT DO THIS ALONE

Unless you are single or living on your own, then you will need to ensure that the people you surround yourself with are on board with your plan, and also offer their support. This is essential if you are prone to cravings and giving in to unhealthy temptations. Ensure that there is an understanding of the health benefits for everyone, which will make it easier to have the on board.

ENJOY YOUR MEALS

Find out how you can enjoy your meals, even with all the changes that you are making. So you are not taking in any more sugar. You can still have a sweet treat by making a smoothie out of your favorite fruit. Instead of feeling terrible about cutting out ice-cream, learn how you can use soya milk, fruit and dark chocolate to create a sinfully delicious dessert. After a long day at work, allow yourself one glass of red wine as you unwind. With the right mindset and motivation, this is one diet that you will enjoy, which is why you can make it last for the long haul.

THE RED MEAT DILEMMA

If you are used to having red meat at almost every meal, this diet may seem challenging. However, all you need to do is change your red meat perspective. On other diets, you may have cheat days where you get to eat whatever you want. This means that you stay on track, looking forward to a cheat day. You can handle your red meat in the same manner. Give yourself some milestones that you need to achieve whilst on this diet. Then you can check on these milestones every two weeks. Each time you meet a milestone, you can reward yourself with a delicious red meat treat. If you do not, you have to pass on this, and work harder at meeting your goals.

THERE ARE NO LIMITS

There are no limits to what you can consume, all you need to do is make some wise sources. Always ask for alternatives if you need any, such as honey instead of sugar, or soya milk instead of dairy. You will be surprised how many establishments, especially if you want to eat out, are able to cater to your unique tastes. In addition, do not eliminate all the things that you love. Just learn how to exercise the right control.

GET RID OF YOUR CAN OPENER

Hopefully, once you start on this diet, you will not need to use your can opener ever again. So why not get rid of it? Your vegetables will be fresh, your meat will be organic and anything that is in a can you can create yourself.

REMEMBER YOUR FIBER

Fiber is often forgotten in diets, yet it has fantastic anti-inflammation properties. Therefore, when you are looking at what you should be eating, particularly your fruit, and vegetables, makes sure that you choose items which are rich in fiber. Furthermore, your first meal of the day should always be fiber rich, as this will make it easier for you to manage in between meals.

Chapter 13: What Is a Tea Cleanse?

A Tea cleanse diet primarily makes use of tea as your main beverage for your daily meals, and should be done in a span of 1 to 3 weeks. According to studies, tea contains Epigalocatechin Gallate (EGCG), a polyphenol that can also be found in most dietary supplements. This boosts metabolism, cleanses the colon, enhances mental performance, as well as improves the mood; that means you will holistically feel better and be healed.

However, this doesn't necessarily mean that tea is the only food product you'll be consuming throughout the day. In fact, even doctors agree that there is no single herb that has the ability to help you lose a lot of weight, as well as cure your health problems just like that.

But, tea is rich in antioxidants and has a special combination of ingredients that somehow prevents diseases, and helps the digestive system do its job properly. Aside from that, tea also aids the ingredients found in healthy foods you eat to give you the right amount of nutrients, and helps your body absorb those nutrients even better.

The 3 R's

The main principle of the tea cleanse diet is Rest, Reduce, and Rebuild. With the help of tea, you'll easily be able to chew your food (more on this later), which means that metabolism would not suffer.

According to Roni DeLuz, a naturpathic doctor, a tea cleanse session should last for 3 weeks, or 21 days. There should be a week-long cleanse for the first 3 weeks, and weekend detox for the next couple of weeks, just so you could maintain your figure and your health would not suffer.

Refresh and Cleanse

This means that it's best to drink tea early in the morning, and before going to bed at night, and that you would also have to drink a few more cups throughout the day, while making sure that you eat nutritious foods, such as oats, fruits, vegetables, brown rice, potatoes, tofu, natural yogurt, unsalted seeds, unsalted nuts, and fish. You also have to hydrate properly by drinking sufficient amounts of water.

And of course, there are also certain food products and drinks that you should stay away from. These include fried and processed foods, alcohol, soda, carbonated drinks, white rice, white bread, and fats.

By only taking what the body needs, you'll be able to make sure that the tea would work properly and would not be inhibited by other ingredients. In time, you'll notice that your organs are functioning a whole lot

better—and you'll feel energetic, instead of being
lethargic all the time.

CHAPTER 14: WHY DO A TEA CLEANSE?

So, how exactly would the tea cleanse diet help you? And why should you do it? Well, here are a number of good reasons.

Tea Metabolizes Fat

First and foremost, tea easily metabolizes fat—while fat is still in the digestive tract. This way, it would easily be broken down into the bloodstream and be turned into energy. This happens with the help of EGCG, which is the most abundant kind of catechin found in tea.

Tea also burns fat because of the right amount of caffeine that it has. Caffeine stimulates thermogenesis, also known as the body's way of generating energy with the help of various food sources. Not only that, tea also has the ability to suppress one's appetite— which means you will easily be satiated and you won't go looking for food all the time!

The Caffeine content of tea is also safe (just around 400 milligrams), which is considered as the acceptable amount of caffeine. In short, it won't give you headaches and palpitations, and also increases the amount of fat-blocking agents in the body, as well!

Tea Improves Memory

Again, thanks to tea's EGCG content, cognition and memory are improved. This is because a phenol called

Noripinepherine is broken down into the bloodstream, and in turn gets to stimulate the brain.

Aside from improving memory, it also improves the body's flight or fight response, and also helps you be more empathetic, too!

Tea Helps You Take in Fewer Calories

With the combination of caffeine, Noripinepherine, and EGCG, you can be sure that tea will only help you take in fewer calories. This means you will feel satiated right away once your body feels like it's getting more calories than necessary.

Emotional hunger happens when you feel a sudden surge of hunger (even though you have just eaten moments ago), when you have certain food cravings, when you keep eating even when you're already full, and when you feel unsatisfied, no matter how much you have eaten.

But, with the help of the tea cleanse diet, this will be prevented from happening because you will always be satiated and so you'll be able to experience real hunger as you should.

Real hunger happens when hunger gets to increase gradually, when you do not feel the need to quickly be full, when you're open to a lot of food options, and when you get to that state where you feel like you're full—and you feel good about it.

And that's so much better, right?

Tea Kills Dangerous Fat

Not all fat are created equal—and the great thing about tea is that it kills dangerous fat so that it would not be able to make its way through your body and so your health would not be in an awful state.

This way, the only fat that will remain in your body are those that are meant to improve the state of your organs, and that would help them function properly.

Tea Is a Great Exercise Aid

It's also best if you would work out while on a diet—and if you think this would be hard, you're wrong. In fact, exercise would be a breeze because you have tea in your system—it helps boost your energy, and helps you work out the right away, so in just 8 weeks or so, you'll be able to lose weight and feel so much better.

As you can see, there are a lot of benefits that you can get simply from drinking tea. In the next chapter, you'll learn how you can do a tea cleanse diet properly.

Chapter 15: How to Do a Tea Cleanse

The tea cleanse diet has two main parts, and these are:

Refresh

Refresh is primarily done in the morning. This is done to help you replace the electrolytes that you have lost, and to gain back some of the vitamins that the body might have lost in the past couple of days. This means you'll have to choose teas that are full of vitamins and antioxidants.

To start, you should first drink a warm-up beverage that's composed of boiled water, lemon slices or lemon juice, and ginger shortly after waking up in the morning. This would wake your organs up, and also help your metabolic levels rise.

Now, after drinking the said warm-up beverage, you can then make your "refresh" tea. This is meant to boost your energy even more and get you started for the day; and could be any of the following:

1. Acai Berry. Acai Berry is the fruit of the Acai palm tree, and contains an impressive amount of antioxidants that refreshes the body thoroughly.

2. Spirulina. Spirulina is a type of freshwater algae that regulates blood sugar levels, and lessens the amount of cholesterol in the body due to its high protein content.

3. Barley Grass. Barley is considered as a major cereal grain, which makes it an amazing source of fiber.

4. Ginseng. Ginseng lowers blood sugar levels and generally boosts the immune system.

Colon Cleanse

The second main part of the tea cleanse diet is called colon cleanse, which means you'll be ridding the colon of toxins. This will also help you become less susceptible to diseases.

The main ingredient you should use here is Senna leaf, which easily prevents constipation and irritable bowel syndrome. It is also effective in the treatment of hemorrhoids, and helps one lose weight fast.

Apart from Senna, other main ingredients you can use include:

1. Nettle Leaf. If you're experiencing urinary tract problems, you can always count on nettle leaf to help you out. It's also used as an astringent, a diuretic, and can prevent and treat ailments of the joints, and alopecia (hair loss) as well.

2. Licorice Root. Licorice prevents stomach inflammation, and keeps the colon free from toxins. It's also great in the prevention of stomach ulcers, colic, and heartburn, and is also used to treat cough, bronchitis, and sore throat. It is said that licorice root may prevent food poisoning, as well.

3. Lemon Grass. Lemon grass is mainly used in the treatment of digestive spasms, as well as achy joints, cough, pain, convulsions, and high blood pressure. It's also used in the prevention of muscle pain. It is used in aromatherapy, as well.

4. Dried Orange Peel. The scent and taste of orange peel is great in soothing the body, and because orange is a citrus fruit, it keeps you protected from various diseases, too.

5. Dandelion. Dandelion has amazing anti-bacterial properties and can also help heal wounds fast. Dandelion is also used in the prevention and treatment of gall stones, kidney stones, and heart weakness. It's a powerful tonic, as well.

Throughout the Day

Apart from Refresh and Colon Cleanse, you also should drink at least 3 to 6 more cups of tea throughout the day. Do this for at least 1 to 3 weeks, together with a proper meal plan which will be discussed later, and you'll surely reach your ideal weight and feel like a lighter, healthier person.

In the next few chapters, you'll learn about different kinds of tea, when you should drink them, and what they can do for you.

Chapter 16: Refresh Teas—the Vitamin-Filled Fat Blockers

Here are some other teas you can use as refresh teas. They're filled with antioxidants, vitamins, minerals, and can surely block fat for you.

Green Tea

Of course, it all starts with green tea!

Green tea rehydrates the body and generally improves immunity.

Green Tea is so popular that in fact, it's already known as a post-workout staple. The thing about green tea is that its anti-oxidant features easily break down fat that help boost energy and hasten the metabolic rate. This way, even if you're not overly active, you can be sure that fat will still be burned—and that you'll eventually lose weight.

Barberry

Meanwhile, there's also a tea called barberry—which is amazing because it prevents fat cells from growing larger.

Barberry is a tea made from the barberry shrub, which is naturally known to prevent weight gain. This also happens even when one is on a high-fat diet.

More so, barberry aids in the prevention of insulin resistance—so it's safe to say that it's good for diabetics, too. Barberry can also increase your energy levels—and when your energy levels are high, it means that you can do a lot in just a short span of time. When you're active, you prevent fat from taking over your body—and that's definitely a good thing!

Japanese Matcha Tea

Learning about the tea ceremony isn't just about appreciating art. It's also about knowing that Japanese tea is actually helpful in the sense that it increases thermogenesis (the use of heat to break fat down, and turn it into energy). From 8 to 10%, thermogenesis reaches 35 to 48% high! It lowers the amount of bad cholesterol, leaving you healthy and protected from heart diseases, too!

Black Tea

Black tea is responsible for reducing fat storage hormones in the body by decreasing cortisol levels. Cortisol is responsible for bad cholesterol and fat formation, and when that is shut down, it follows that you will lose fat in your body, too.

It's best to drink black tea when you are stressed because it's also during that time that adrenaline is able to break fat down, and release fat into your system to turn them into energy.

When adrenaline and cortisol work together, the body is able to break more fat down—and in turn, prevent the body from consuming more calories, too.

Rooibos

The best thing about rooibos tea is that it inhibits fat cell formation. You see, when there are no fat cells, there's also a very low chance that you'd gain lots of fat, in the first place. By drinking Rooibos tea, you get to prevent fat cell formation by up to 22%!

Aside from that, rooibos also prevents stress, thanks to its unique combination of flavonoids. This way, one's hunger is also suppressed—which leads to fat-burning, as well.

Pu-erh (Fermented Green Tea)

This tea is the kind of tea that's fermented and then rolled into blocks, which can help lower triglyceride compounds. These triglycerides are basically the dangerous kind of fat that's found in one's blood.

Aside from that, Pu-erh also lowers the amount of abdominal fat, even in high-fat diets—which is definitely a good thing!

White Tea

White tea is the type of tea that's naturally sun-dried, which makes it full of anti-oxidants. The compounds found in white tea are then able to block the formation of fat cells, as well as break fat down and turn it into energy instead.

Its antioxidants, meanwhile, are able to trigger fat release from the cells and help the liver turn the fat into energy, which, of course, is beneficial to the body.

CHAPTER 17: COLON CLEANSE TEAS—TEAS THAT RID THE COLON OF TOXINS, AND HELP YOU SLEEP BETTER!

As mentioned earlier, colon cleanse is the second major part of the tea cleanse diet. It should be done shortly before going to bed, and with that in mind, here are the teas you should have in your pantry:

Garlic Tea

Garlic may prove to be somehow challenging for you to drink, but the thing with garlic tea is that it strengthens the body's detoxification process. Your body would be able to easily flush toxins away.

Garlic also strengthens the immune system and protects you against a lot of diseases, making life even better for you.

Cayenne Pepper Tea

Since it is naturally spicy, you can expect cayenne pepper tea to curb your appetite, with the help of capsaicin, and also to flush those toxins while elevating your mood.

Aside from being a good detox aid, it also energizes you a whole lot—making it one of the best teas you can keep.

If you feel like it's a little too hot for you, you can always try drinking it with lemon slices.

Cilantro Tea

Cilantro not only spices up your dishes, you can also use it for detoxification purposes.

The thing with cilantro is that it breaks down food so nutrients would easily be released without disrupting your digestive processes. Cilantro is also considered to be highly curative.

Burdock Root Tea

While not as popular as its contemporaries, burdock root is a liver tonic that has the ability to detoxify a lot. A highly functioning liver regulates digestive processes, which means that there would be less toxic buildup in your digestive tract. Burdock also purifies the blood and strengthens the immune system—and when holistic healing is promoted, you know you're drinking a good thing.

Chicory Tea

By drinking chicory tea, it's like you're hitting two birds with one stone because it not only cleanses the body, it hastens metabolic rate, as well.

It is best to drink chicory tea before a meal because it can get digestive juices going, which would then be responsible for the easy breakdown of food. This tea also helps you get all the nutrients you can get from what you have been eating.

Gymnema Sylvestre Tea

This is a Chinese herb that is known for being able to regulate blood glucose levels, and can also reverse the effect of digestive disorders.

More so, it cleanses the liver and the colon—and makes sure that you are protected against diabetes.

Ginger Tea

Ginger is considered to be one the highest cleansing teas out there. Sure, the taste may be a bit sharp, but it's so beneficial it really does not matter anymore. Besides, you could always tame it down with the help of lemon slices, you know?

Fenugreek Tea

It's best to drink Fenugreek tea when you're feeling a little bit under the weather and you feel like your digestive system is suffering. It helps keep you from getting bloated, and also helps prevent indigestion from happening.

Inflammation is reduced and high blood pressure is prevented—what more could you ask

for?

Guduchi Tea

Guduchi has amazing restorative properties that improve organ function and also keep the skin glowing and healthy at all times.

Manjistha Tea

Did you know that in order to eliminate toxins, you should also take care of your skin? Well, this is because the skin is the body's largest organ so if you do not take care of it, it wouldn't be able to help the liver in flushing those toxins away.

Manjistha has a lot of medicinal properties, especially for menstruating women. It's best for menstruating women to help keep them calm during that dreaded time of the month, so they could get rid of more toxins and keep their bodies safe!

Red Clover Tea

Red clover tea is able to fight free radicals because it contains a lot of antioxidants, and also makes sure that your body would not play host to organisms and parasites that could cause diseases. Always go for organic red clover tea.

Milk Thistle Tea

Milk thistle can help your liver work the best way it can.

You see, detox diets work best when you have something that can really keep the liver safe, and make sure that it does its job of producing the right amount of digestive juices. Milk thistle regulates digestive processes, too!

Triphala Tea

Triphala treats constipation and stimulates bowel movements, which means that your colon would be healthy and clean. It's also important to take care of the colon because if you don't, it could reintroduce those toxins back again—and that's not what you want to happen.

Yellow Dock Tea

Yellow dock takes care of both the colon and the liver, which means that toxins are easily eliminated, and digestion is improved—definitely making you feel like your best self ever.

Turmeric Tea

Turmeric tea breaks toxins down and flushes them away for good. It also helps the liver produce more bile so that your body would be clean at all times, and so digestive processes would easily be regulated.

Wormwood Tea

And finally, don't forget wormwood tea.

This helps the liver produce more bile, and makes sure that digestive processes would not be stagnant. It's also best to drink this daily, even after the 3 weeks of the diet.

CHAPTER 18: TEAS TO DRINK THROUGHOUT THE DAY

And of course, you should also make sure that you have the right ingredients at hand so that you'd also be able to make tea throughout the day. Remember, you need at least 3 to 6 cups!

Here are the said teas:

Oolong Tea

More than 150% of fat is burned, and metabolism is enhanced triple time by oolong tea!

Aside from enhancing metabolism, oolong tea also prevents the body from absorbing more fat than it can handle. In just 2 weeks, fat is blocked by up to 50% already, thanks to natural oxidation process!

Oolong also increases the body's plasma adiponectin levels that are responsible for protecting the body against obesity. You can either make this in a matter or 5 to 30 minutes; the longer, the more flavor is maximized.

Rose Tea

Not only does it smell good, it actually tastes great, too!

Rose tea boosts metabolism as it contains a combination of Vitamins A, B3, C, D, and E. Not only that, it also keeps the body safe from infections, prevents constipation, and is highly therapeutic.

Use petals and buds to make tea, but make sure to clean the petals first with the help of boiling water. Steep for 2 to 3 minutes.

Peppermint Tea

You know what's great about peppermint tea? Well, it actually helps your body gain more control when it comes to the things you eat. It helps you keep satiated, and taps EGCG to do its job, therefore enhancing metabolism.

You can make peppermint tea by using the leaves of the peppermint plant. Use either fresh or dried leaves and steep for at least 4 to 5 minutes.

Star Anise Tea

Native to China, star anise treats stomach upset and diarrhea—and also helps suppress the appetite.

To get maximum effects, steep a star anise pod for at least 10 minutes. Feel free to blend it with other ingredients or teas because drinking it alone might be a little too bitter for your taste.

Make some by using coffee grinder or by steeping the tea in squash gourd!

Feiyan Tea

Fat that is accumulated by the body could be reduced with the help of Feiyan Tea.

You see, this tea is made of a combination of plants, such as jasmine, lotus, and vegetable sponge that contain no chemical elements. This means that there would be no side effects, and that you can lose up to 8 lbs in the first week of the diet alone, especially if you drink this on the first night of the diet itself.

Not only does it boost metabolism, it detoxifies the body, too!

Porangaba Tea

Mostly found in South America, Porangaba is known as Brazil's special weight loss potion. It has just the right amount of caffeine that could hasten metabolic rate and prevent fat from ruining the body.

More so, Porangaba suppresses the appetite, but does not destroy the organs as it is a natural diuretic. Drink some 30 minutes before each meal and you're all set!

Yerba Mate

Good cholesterol levels are stimulated with the help of Yerba Mate. Enzymes that break down bad cholesterol are tapped with the help of polyphenols and antioxidants that are found in Yerba Mate.

CHAPTER 19: SAMPLE 1 WEEK MEAL PLAN

To give you a better idea about how you could incorporate teas in your daily diet, here's a sample 1 week meal plan that would give you some clarity—and some great meal ideas, too!

Day 1

Breakfast

Cream Cheese and Salmon Bagel

Barley Grass Tea

Morning Snack

1 cup blueberries

Oolong Tea

Lunch

Veggie and Mushroom Stir Fry

Porangaba Tea

Afternoon Snack

½ Grapefruit

Peppermint Tea

Dinner

Chicken Fajitas

Cilantro Tea

Day 2

Breakfast

Cereal and Toast

Matcha Tea

Morning Snack

2 Nectarines

Rose Tea

Lunch

Baked Cod

Yerba Mate

Afternoon Snack

Celery Sticks with Hummus

Feiyan Tea

Dinner

Bean and Chili Casserole

Milk Thistle Tea

Day 3

Breakfast

Boiled Egg, Fruit, Toast

Acai Berry Tea

Morning Snack

½ cup plum + ½ cup strawberries

Black Tea

Lunch

Italian Bread Salad

Star Anise Tea

Afternoon Snack

Carrot Sticks + Hummus

Oolong Tea

Dinner

Chicken Fillets with Sundried Tomatoes

Garlic Tea

Day 4

Breakfast

Fruits, Nuts, and Yogurt

Spirulina Tea

Morning Snack

½ cup pineapple + Nori Chips

Barberry Tea

Lunch

Mango and Zucchini Kebabs

Feiyan Tea

Afternoon Snack

Sunflower Seeds + Celery Sticks

Peppermint Tea

Dinner

Smoked Mackerel Pasta

Fenugreek Tea

Day 5

Breakfast

Peanut Butter and Banana Toast

Barley Grass Tea

Morning Snack

5 Dried Prunes + Low Fat Cottage Cheese

White Tea

Lunch

Beans on Toast

Yerba Mate

Afternoon Snack

Pears + Almonds

Rose Tea

Dinner

Vegetable Omelette

Cayenne Pepper Tea

Day 6

Breakfast

Cereal, Banana, and Apricot

Rooibos Tea

Morning Snack

½ cup green grapes + fruit yogurt

Barberry Tea

Lunch

Chili Con Carne

Porangaba Tea

Afternoon Snack

5 Almonds + ½ cup green grapes

Oolong Tea

Dinner

Chicken and Noodles

Red Clover Tea

Day 7

Breakfast

Asparagus and Eggs

Green Tea

Morning Snack

5 dried prunes + carrot sticks

White Tea

Lunch

Egg and Cress Sandwich

Rose Tea

Afternoon Snack

½ cup plum + ½ cup strawberries

Peppermint Tea

Dinner

Baked Salmon with Peppers

Cayenne Pepper Tea

As you can see, this meal plan has the right amount of protein, fruits, and tea that would make a great difference in your health! Make this your guide, and help yourself create creative and nutritious meal plans soon!

CHAPTER 20: OTHER REMINDERS

Finally, here are some other things that you should keep in mind while on the tea cleanse diet—to make it work even better!

1. Boost Circulation. In order to easily turn fat into energy, you do have to boost circulation. Do so by exercising. You see, you do have to take care of your lymph nodes by making sure lympathic fluid flows steadily—and deep-breathing exercises as well as jump-roping could help you out with this. It would be nice if you'd find time to laugh, too—that would definitely drive the stress away!

2. Chew Starchy Vegetables and Beans Slowly. Potatoes, sweet potatoes, yams, cauliflower, broccoli, and other cruciferous vegetables could make you gassy—so take your time in chewing them. By eating beans regularly, your body gets immune to the gassy feeling—just make sure that you add small amounts only.

3. Chew Your Food Slowly. You know, most fast eaters end up with bloated bellies because they don't take time to chew their food. The thing with not chewing food slowly is that you end up sucking too much air which could then lead to bloating. So, just take your time. Remember, eating isn't a race—make sure that you enjoy your food, and that you eat properly.

4. Don't Drink Too Much Carbonated Drinks. Carbonated drinks (even low-cal/diet ones) just trap gas inside your body, so if you're not a big fan of water, you can spruce it up a bit by adding lime, lemon, or orange—to turn it into flavored water. Peppermint tea could also help, as well.

5. Eat 5 to 6 Small Meals Instead of 2 to 3 Big Meals. Doing so would prevent you from feeling bloated, and would make it easy for your body to digest and metabolize what you have eaten. Plus, when you eat small meals, you get to prevent yourself from feeling hungry over and over again.

6. Go to the Sauna! You could sweat it out at the sauna—which will easily rid your body of toxins, or brush the skin with sugar or salt. It would also be best if you could switch to all-organic beauty products. You do not need any artificial elements in your skin!

7. Hydrate Yourself. At times when emotional hunger arises, do yourself a favor, and keep yourself hydrated. This way, toxins would be flushed away, and digestive processes would be regulated. You can also try working on a project, or going out just so you could distract yourself from eating more than you should. It's not only the liver and kidneys that you should think of; you have to give your kidney the time of day, too! Make sure that while on the tea cleanse diet, you have to go to the bathroom to pee at least once every hour, and that

you drink 6 to 8 glasses of water a day. It's always best to stay hydrated!

8. Limit Sodium Intake. Sodium is abundant in processed foods (i.e. junk foods, chips, soda, etc.) so it's important to minimize your intake of those. Another good tip is to make sure that you read food labels properly. Choose those that say "low-sodium" or "sodium-free". It's important to make sure that you do not take more than 500mg of sodium in a day.

9. Look for Sugar-Free Foods. Bloating is also caused by taking too much alcohol and sugar-laden foods, so make sure that you don't take more than 2 to 3 servings of sugary foods per day.

10. Stay Away from Chewing Gum. Chewing gum also makes you suck in more air than necessary. Sometimes, it's hard to stay away from chewing gum, though, because it's a habit of many, but what you can do is just choose other healthy food, when you're in need of a good snack. Try low-fat popcorn, fruits, and vegetables instead.

11. Try Probiotics. Probiotics are simply good bacteria that keep the immune system healthy, and prevent bloating by regulating digestive process. They also regulate the amount of good bacteria in the body, as well.

12. Work the Lungs Out. In order to strengthen the lungs, you have to work them out, too. You could do

this by doing deep-breathing exercises. Visualize how you'd inhale all the nutrients you need, as well as how you'd exhale toxins away. These will certainly help.

As mentioned earlier, teas won't work on their own. It's best that you aid them with the right kinds of food, and also make sure that you get to exercise, and you do not let yourself get dehydrated or stressed. This way, the tea cleanse diet would really work for you!

CHAPTER 21: RECIPES

Detoxing doesn't mean your tea should taste like water. There are a lot of recipes you can use to enhance your tea. However, you may not know any of these.

If so, there is no need to stress. In this chapter, I will share some recipes to get you going. When you are done with these, you can look for more online.

1. BOSTON ICED TEA

For those who love iced tea, you will love this recipe. And I bet you will be turning to it daily. Making it better, it has Cranberry juice added, which helps with urinary tract infections, cancer, kidney stones, and heart disease (Recipe courtesy allrecipes.com)

Ingredients

- 1 gallon of water

- 1 cup sugar (or less depending on your needs)

- 10-15 tea bags

- 1 can of frozen cranberry juice concentrate

Instructions

- Heat water in a large pot until it boils

- Add sugar and stir for a minute

- Add the tea bags in. Leave them to steep for at least 5 minutes

- Stir in the cranberry juice concentrate.

- Serve with ice

2. HONEY LEMON TEA

The best part of this recipe is that it needs less that 5 minutes of your time. Also, it has lemon juice and honey, both of which are super foods. As if not enough, the resulting tea is low in calories.

However, although I've included sugar on the ingredients, you can do without it (Recipe courtesy allrecipes.com)

Ingredients

- 1 tbs lemon juice

- 2 tbs honey

- 1 cup water

- Sugar, to taste

Instructions

- Boil water

- Add lemon juice, honey, and sugar into a mug

- Pour boiling water into the mug and stir.

3. Good Ol' Alabama Sweet Tea

For all those with sweet teeth, this is a recipe to save (Recipe courtesy allrecipes.com)

Ingredients

- 1 cup sugar

- 1/2 gallon water

- 1 tray ice cubes

- 3 family sized tea bags of orange Pekoe tea

- 3 cups cold water

Instructions

- Heat water in a large pot and kill heat just when the water is about to boil.

- Place your tea bags in the pot and let them steep for 5 minutes. Meanwhile, you should pour the sugar into a pitcher

- After the 5 minutes, remove the teabags from the pot and bring back the heat till the water begins to boil.

- You should then pour the boiling water into the pitcher and stir till most of the sugar is dissolved.

- Fill half of the pitcher with ice and stir

- Add cold water to the mixture and stir.

4. MINT TEA PUNCH

This is another recipe any tea lover will enjoy. Just like with the others before, this won't require you to stand in the kitchen for too long. But in the end, you will have 14 cups of tea.(Recipe courtesy food.com)

Ingredients

- 5 cups boiling water

- 7 cups water

- 1 cup sugar

- 1 can frozen orange juice concentrate

- 1 can frozen lemon juice concentrate

- 5 regular sized tea bags

- 8 mint sprigs, crushed

Instructions

- Put mint sprigs and tea bags in a large pitcher and pour boiling water over them

- Cover with a lid and let them steep for 5 minutes

- Stir in your sugar and let it steep for another 5 minutes

- Remove tea bags, then pour the mixture through a strainer to get rid of the mint sprigs

- Stir in the water, lemon, and orange juice concentrates

5.Smooth Sweet Tea

Here is another recipe for all those who love sweet tea (Recipe courtesy allrecipes.com)

Ingredients

- 1 pinch baking soda

- 2 cups boiling water

- 6 tea bags

- 3/4 cup white sugar

- 6 cups cold water

Instructions

- Sprinkle a pinch of salt into a 64 ounce, heat proof, glass pitcher.

- Add boiling water as well as the tea bags

- Cover with a lid and allow for a steeping time of 15 minutes

- Remove tea bags and stir in sugar

- Add cold water and refrigerate until cold

6. Iced Green Tea with Ginger and Mint

Here is another one of my favorite tea recipes (Recipe courtesy of epicurious.com).

Ingredients

- 3 ounces ginger unpeeled and sliced

- 1 cup mint leaves

- 6 green tea bags

- 1/2 cup honey

- 2 tbs lemon juice

- 6 cups water

Instructions

Add ginger and the 6 cups of water in a large pan and boil

- Kill the heat, then add mint leaves and the tea bags

- Cover with a lid and let the mixture steep for 15 minutes

- Strain the liquid into a pitcher

- Stir in honey and lemon juice

- Serve with ice cubes and mint leaves

7. PUFFED WILD RICE GREEN TEA

Wild rice is superior to white rice in terms of healthy benefits. And it gets even healthier when you couple it with green tea. Here is the recipe (Recipe courtesy of canadianliving.com).

Ingredients

- 1/4 cup wild rice

- 1 cup green tea leaves (e.g., Japanese Sencha)

Instructions

- Heat a nonstick skillet over high heat

- Add wild rice and toast for 30 seconds, keep shaking.

- Pour the wild rice into a bowl and let it cool

- Mix green tea leaves with the rice

- Store the mixture in an airtight jar

8. Spiced Tea Mix

If you are a fan of healthy spices, this is your recipe. And it's easy to prepare (Recipe courtesy of allrecipes.com).

Ingredients

- 1 package lemon-flavored ice tea mix

- 2 packages orange-flavored drink mix, (e.g., Tang)

- 1 1/3 tbs ground cinnamon

- 2 tsps ground cloves

Instructions

- Mix all ingredients well

- Store in an airtight container

- When serving, stir 1 1/2 tsp of the mixture into 1 cup hot water

9. HOT CHAI LATTE

This recipe is delicious. No wonder it is a hit with many people (Recipe courtesy of allrecipes.com).

Ingredients

- 1 cup milk

- 1 cup water

- 3 whole cloves

- 1 cinnamon stick

- 1 large strip of orange peel

- 4 tsps white sugar

- 2 tsps black tea leaves

- 3 whole black peppercorns

- 1 pinch ground nutmeg

Instructions

- Warm milk and water over medium heat

- Add the rest of the ingredients

- Let the mixture boil, after which you should reduce heat to medium-low

- Simmer till it darkens to your liking

- Strain the liquid and serve

10. RUSSIAN TEA

Although Russians are known for their obsession with Vodka, they are also good at making tea. And you can prove that with this recipe (Recipe courtesy of allrecipes.com).

Ingredients

- 1 cup instant tea powder

- 2 cups orange-flavored drink mix (e.g. Tang)

- 1 package powdered lemonade mix

- 2 cups white sugar

- 2 tsps ground cinnamon

- 1/2 tsps ground cloves

Instructions

- Mix all the ingredients in a large bowl

- Store the contents in an airtight jar

- When serving, take 3 or 4 tablespoons of the mixture and combine with 1 cup of water. Note that the water can be cold or warm depending on your preferences.

GINGER-CERASSE TEA

This tea recipe requires infusion. The best way to get the nutrients from Cerasse leaves is to boil it. Native to Africa and the Middle East, Cerasse leaves can be found at your local market. Cerasse works in eliminating toxins from the body. It is also great for promoting digestive health and improving liver function. This recipe makes 1 to 2 servings.

Ingredients:

-2 cups of water

-2-inch slice of ginger root, peeled and cut into thin slices

-2 teaspoons of honey

-Handful of Cerasse leaves with the vines intact

Directions:

1.Boil 2 cups of water in a kettle over medium high heat.

2.Once boiling, add ginger slices and Cerasse leaves with vines.

3.Reduce heat and cover to simmer for 10 to 15 minutes. Set aside to cool.

4.Strain the mixture and pour into a cup or glass. Stir in the honey and enjoy!

TAHEEBO TEA

The Taheebo tree, which can grow as high as 90 meters, is found in Brazil and Argentina. Its bark, named Pau d'Arco, is used for making tea. Health food stores sell Pau d'Arco in its loose form. According to folklore, tea made from Taheebo possesses anti-microbial properties. This is responsible for Taheebo's cleansing and strengthening abilities. Other benefits of this tea include strengthening the immune system and inhibiting candida. It also acts as a general body tonic and detoxifier.

There is something refreshing about Taheebo tea. It can taste slightly bitter which is why some people like to add either honey or maple syrup to the concoction. Taheebo tea can be enjoyed either hot or cold. You may want to try it with a slice of lemon served on ice.

Why Taheebo Tea is good for you

Taheebo has been widely used by South American tribes and the ancient Incas because of its medicinal properties. It is believed to help treat various diseases.

The plant can be applied internally or externally. In addition to its anti-microbial properties, Taheebo also possesses antibiotic, antibacterial, antiviral and anti-inflammatory properties amongst other benefits. Here are more reasons why drinking this tea is good for you.

1. Improve Blood Health

This tea promotes blood health in many ways. One, it assists in purifying blood. In fact, it has been used as a blood cleanser for thousands of years. It does not only purify the blood, it also acts as a general body detoxifier which means it helps make your entire body toxin free. As a result, you become stronger and healthier. Two, it improves red blood cell count. Three, the tea also promotes healthy blood circulation.

2. Improve Digestion

Because of its laxative properties, Taheebo tea is effective in the regulation of bowel movement and stimulation of digestion at the same time. It not only helps prevent constipation and flatulence problems but can also assist in weight reduction.

3. Strengthen Immunity

Also known as Lapacho, Taheebo acts as a natural antibiotic. It has powerful antioxidants that can help in preventing diseases and fighting off free radicals. Drinking this tea regularly will help to keep sore throats, fevers, colds, the flu and other common diseases at bay.

4. Treat and Prevent Infections

As mentioned previously, Taheebo can reduce candida overgrowth and prevent yeast infections. It is also good for treating parasitic and fungal infections especially when applied directly to the skin. Taken internally, Taheebo tea can also be an effective treatment for gonorrhea and syphilis amongst other sexually transmitted diseases.

5. Reduce Inflammations

People suffering from inflammation can also benefit from drinking Taheebo in its tea form. Its anti-inflammatory properties work effectively in reducing prostate and bladder inflammations. It has even been used as an effective treatment for arthritis pain and symptoms.

6. Treat AIDS, Cancer and Chronic Diseases

Taheebo tea is also used as alternative treatment for AIDS. For this purpose, Taheebo is typically combined with licorice, Echinacea and Spirulina. It is also believed to help treat and prevent cancer. As a matter of fact, Taheebo tea has been promoted as an anti-cancer agent for many years. It may also help with chronic diseases including Parkinson's disease, lupus and psoriasis.

Aside from the health benefits mentioned above, Taheebo tea contains anti-aging properties. It can also be used as a natural remedy for ulcers, toothache, varicose veins, back pain, liver disease, diabetes, gastritis, leukemia, impotence and malaria among other diseases.

How to make Taheebo Tea

You will need the following:

-3 tablespoons of dried Taheebo bark

-About 10 cups of water

Directions:

1.Pour 10 cups of water in a pot.

2.Add the 3 tablespoons of dried Taheebo bark.

3.Bring to a boil for approximately 5 minutes, over high heat.

4.Reduce heat to simmer for 15 minutes.

5.Set it aside to cool before straining.

You can enjoy the tea hot. Just add a slice of lemon and honey. Then, you can store the leftover tea in the fridge by pouring the pot's contents in a glass container. The Taheebo tea can be enjoyed throughout the day.

Additional Tips and Reminders in Making Taheebo Tea

When making taheebo tea, it is best to use glass, porcelain or steel pots. Avoid using pots and containers made of plastic or aluminum. Using aluminum or plastic pots and containers will affect the flavor, so it is best to avoid using them. If you are not accustomed to drinking tea, it may taste a little bitter. Otherwise, Taheebo tea has a mild flavor. If you add any additional ingredients, the tea will adapt to that flavor. For example, you can boil the Taheebo bark with crushed blueberries and it will taste like blueberry tea.

Feel free to add honey, but avoid adding sugar. From preparation, the tea can last up to 4 days at room temperature or up to 8 days when refrigerated. You can mix 3 tablespoons or up to 5 tablespoons of Taheebo bark to 10 cups of water. To keep the integrity of the tea, it is also recommended that you use either purified or distilled water. This is to make sure that your tea is free from additives and to maintain its flavor. In fact, using purified or distilled water is just good tea practice for all of your weight loss, detox concoctions.

Taheebo bark is tannin rich. Your body will absorb these tannins much more efficiently with lemon. Even a small amount of freshly squeezed lemon juice can help you maximize the benefits of this powerful plant.

Side Effects and Precautions

The recommended dosage is at two cups of Taheebo tea per day. If you are treating a condition, you can consume up to 8 cups but not more. Speak with your health care practitioner for suggestions regarding precise medicinal quantities. This tea is toxic to parasites, cancer cells, bacteria, viruses and other bad microorganisms. It is not harmful to healthy cells. However, it is best to keep your consumption to a minimum. As much as possible, you must stick to the recommended dosage. Otherwise, you may suffer from side effects.

Consuming too much of this tea may cause mild dizziness, nausea, diarrhea and vomiting. Be mindful however, that some of these side effects are a natural result of detoxification. When you consume the tea, your urine may turn pink and that is normal.

Pregnant women are advised against taking the tea. Taheebo tea acts as an anticoagulant, which is why it is not advised for people taking medicine with the same effect, or for people about to undergo surgery.

DANDELION TEA

Dandelion is another herb used for medicinal purposes. The leaves and roots are typically dried to make tea. The herb is also a common ingredient for soups and salads. Dandelion roots can also be roasted to make coffee substitute, and many enjoy dandelion wine.

Why Dandelion Tea is good for you

This Dandelion tea can boost digestive function. It works as a laxative. At the same time, it helps increase urine production. Therefore, you can tell it is absolutely amazing for detoxification.

How to make Dandelion Tea

On its own, Dandelion can make an effective weight loss drink. Here's how to make a basic Dandelion tea. Be warned however that Dandelion tea is not for the faint hearted. It has a bitter taste, which may take some time to get used to. Adding a teaspoon of honey to a cup of Dandelion tea may improve the taste.

Ingredients:

-1 tablespoon of dried Dandelion roots

-1 cup of water

Directions:

1.Heat water and add dried Dandelion roots.

2.Allow the mixture to steep for 5 minutes.

1.*This drink can be enjoyed hot or cold.

ULTIMATE DANDELION DETOX TEA

This detox recipe can help jumpstart weight loss by eliminating excess water weight from your body. It is easy to make and has an interesting flavor too. This recipe makes one pitcher.

Ingredients:

-60 ounces of water (7.5 cups)

-1 to 2 teaspoons of dried dandelion root

-2 tablespoons of freshly squeezed lemon juice

-1 tablespoon of cranberry juice, sugar-free

Directions:

1.Boil water in a kettle over medium high heat. Set aside to cool for 3 minutes.

2.Add dried dandelion root to the hot water. Allow it to steep for 5 minutes.

3.Strain the tea mixture and pour into a pitcher.

4.Stir in the freshly squeezed lemon juice and cranberry juice.

*You can enjoy this concoction throughout the day. Continue to make and drink this tea recipe for a week to lose excess water weight.

Additional Tips and Reminders in Making Dandelion Tea

In place of dried Dandelion leaves and roots, which can be purchased at health food stores, you may use Dandelion teabags. To maximize the benefits however, using the dried Dandelion parts is recommended.

Side Effects and Precautions

Dandelion tea is generally safe with no known side effects. There are no harmful effects in consuming dandelion either as tea or as food, as long as you do not have it in excessive amounts.

While it is considered safe to consume the tea, pregnant and breastfeeding women should still avoid using it. In addition, people with known allergies to ragweed may experience the same reaction to Dandelion tea. In which case, it is best to avoid it.

CELERY SEED TEA

You know celery seeds from potato salad. However, did you know these seeds are also great home remedies? They possess anti-bacterial properties that work to treat gout, headaches and urinary tract disorders. They are also effective against kidney problems. As a matter of fact, celery seed tea is a traditional remedy. Many herbalists today stand by its medicinal benefits.

Why Celery Seed Tea is good for you

For the purpose of losing weight, you'll be interested to know that Celery seed tea acts as a natural diuretic. Just like Dandelion tea, it works by increasing urine production to flush out toxins from the body. And, it's just as good at getting rid of excess water weight.

The seeds are rich in natural organic sodium and potassium, which assist in the elimination of waste buildup in the kidneys, bowels and skin. They also have many healthy fatty acids! Lastly, Celery seed tea promotes a healthy balance between acid and alkaline in the body.

How to make Celery Seed Tea

Celery seed tea is prepared by crushing or grinding the seeds, then steeping the powder in boiling water.

Here's how you can make your own tea. This recipe makes up to 3 cups.

Ingredients:

-3 cups of water

-1 tablespoon of crushed or ground celery seeds

Directions:

1.Boil water in a kettle over medium high heat.

2.Once boiling, turn off heat and toss in the celery seed powder.

3.Let it steep and cool for 10 or up to 20 minutes, strain.

Additional Tips and Reminders in Making Celery Seed Tea

The amount of minerals that you get from the tea depends on how long you let it steep. Celery seeds are available from your local health food stores. You may find garden seeds too but do not make the mistake of using them. Rather than helping you eliminate toxic waste, those garden seeds are toxic themselves. They are cured with a bunch of chemicals and the last thing you want is to use them as tea.

The above recipe makes 3 cups of tea. You can have Celery seed tea in place of Dandelion tea. As compared to the bitter Dandelion, this Celery tea has a milder taste. You can have as much as 3 cups a day.

Side Effects and Precautions

Consuming Celery Seed tea is generally safe. However because of it may lead to uterine contractions, it is not advisable for pregnant women. In addition, the tea may be beneficial to the kidneys, but anyone suffering from kidney problems should consult with a health practitioner first before using this as a remedy.

WATERMELON SEED TEA

Who doesn't find watermelon refreshing, especially during the hot summer months? The fruit is an excellent source of antioxidants and minerals. It keeps us hydrated. While we love eating watermelon, most of us find the seeds bothersome. We spit them out and forget about them. Little do we know, they can save us from pesky belly fat!

Why Watermelon Seed Tea is good for you

Like other fruit seeds, watermelon seeds offer a mild laxative effect. They also promote digestion and are a highly effective remedy for constipation.

Tea concocted from watermelon seeds promotes kidney health. It works to detoxify the body and reduce toxic waste build up. For centuries, watermelon seed tea has been relied on for detoxifying the kidneys and eliminating kidney stones.

The cleansing effect of this tea is quite remarkable. The seeds are low in calories but they provide a good amount of energy, which can spell the difference in your physical performance. Like the fruit, the seeds are an excellent source of antioxidants, zinc and magnesium. Other benefits include improving blood pressure and treating urinary tract infections.

How to make Watermelon Seed Tea

Here is the basic watermelon seed tea recipe. This recipe makes one serving.

Ingredients:

-1 1/2 cups of water

-1 tablespoon of watermelon seeds

Directions:

1.Boil water in a kettle over medium high heat.

2.Once boiling, reduce the heat and toss the watermelon seeds into the kettle. Cover and simmer for 30 minutes.

3.Remove from heat and allow it to steep for an hour.

4.Strain the mixture and serve.

*To sweeten the tea drink, you may add crushed watermelon fruit or stir in a teaspoon of honey for every cup. Never resort to using sugar. That will defeat the purpose of cleansing.

Additional Tips and Reminders for Making Watermelon Seed Tea

It doesn't matter what kind of watermelon seeds you use, chopped or ground work the same. You can even buy a whole watermelon and collect the seeds. Grind or chop them yourself.

Although it is fine to make big batches of other teas, it is best to make a fresh cup of watermelon seed tea each time. You will maximize the tea's benefits from a freshly brewed cup. The recommended dosage is one cup a day, 3 times weekly.

For a more efficient cleansing, you can drink as much as 3 to 4 cups a day. However, do not exceed the limit of 40 grams of watermelon seeds daily. Have your first cup first thing in the morning. It is best taken on an empty stomach. Take another cup 30 minutes after you have breakfast and another after the two other meals of the day at the same time interval. With this dosage, you can perform the treatment two times a week.

Side Effects and Precautions

There are no known side effects for consuming watermelon seed tea except when you consume too much. Overconsumption of this tea may lead to vomiting, nausea, gas formation and indigestion. Elderly cleansers should be especially mindful of their dosage. That's because the intestinal tract becomes weaker with age, which means the side effects of consuming too much tea may also be worse for them.

Although watermelon seed tea promotes kidney health, those already suffering from kidney problems must consult with a doctor first before using this as a remedy. It is also not advisable for people with known allergies to watermelon.

CONCLUSION

This is a diet that is not a diet, rather, it has clearly revealed itself to be a way of life that will change your life. You can expect to inevitably lose some weight the moment you start to eat right. Once you have lost this weight, it will become easier to maintain a healthy body weight for the rest of your life. However, that is not the goal of the anti-inflammatory diet.

Making the changes to your diet and adopting the principles of the anti-inflammatory diet will not result in immediate change. However, in a relatively short period of time, it will become clear that this diet has substantial benefits, as you find that any troubling and uncomfortable symptoms you experienced begin to dissipate. Thus, you will also become less dependent on conventional medicine.

At the core of the anti-inflammatory diet is one premise which states that you need to eat healthy foods if you want to live a long life. This means that of the three main food groups which are carbohydrates, proteins and fats, you must consume healthy alternatives which are rich in nutrient. Eating processed foods can seriously increase the possibility of inflammation.

The right balance can lead to a complete change in your life, without you needing to go through deprivation or lack. Indeed, this is one diet plan that you and your family should take on today. Do not waste another moment. Get started with this plan.

www.ingramcontent.com/pod-product-compliance
Lightning Source LLC
Chambersburg PA
CBHW062134020426
42335CB00013B/1210